UP FROM SUICIDE

and Other Short Stories

IRENE PIERCE DUNN

Up From Suicide
Copyright © 2020 by Irene Pierce Dunn

All rights reserved. No part of this publication may be reproduced, distributed, or transmitted in any form or by any means, including photocopying, recording, or other electronic or mechanical methods, without the prior written permission of the author, except in the case of brief quotations embodied in critical reviews and certain other non-commercial uses permitted by copyright law.

Holy Bible quotes are from the King James Version.

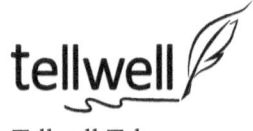

Tellwell Talent
www.tellwell.ca

ISBN
978-0-2288-4116-6 (Paperback)
978-0-2288-7584-0 (eBook)

CONTENTS

SPLINTERED PUZZLE PIECES 1
DADDY'S NOT HOME 5
PRETEND YOU ARE ASLEEP 17
FIFTY-TWO PICK-UP / TRAFFICKED 27
MA KATE 33
MY MOTHER MY MUDDLE 45
MAXIMUM GROWTH 53
DEEP IMPRESSIONS 59
WHEN THE MIND CALLS FOR TIME OUT 69
UP FROM SUICIDE 77
AND GOD LAUGHED 89
AMENDS 95
EXERCISING DEMOCRACY 107
BOBBY 117
THE AMERICAN SCREAM 123

THE IMPACT OF 9/11	133
OVERCOMING SMOKE	141
PRETEND YOU ARE NORMAL	147
THE PRESENT	157
GRATITUDE	169
ABBA FATHER	173

SPLINTERED PUZZLE PIECES

When I was in my early twenties, I felt like a piece of puzzle that did not belong in any box. Wherever I went, the feeling persisted that I did not belong or fit in. The puzzle piece that belonged nowhere was an apt description of exactly how I felt. Two decades later, I was mulling over several boxes of my twelve-year-old son's puzzles with missing pieces. I had the great idea all of a sudden that it really did not matter if the puzzle pieces were all mixed up. Why not just glue them together and create a masterpiece sculpture? Of course, I was too stoned on marijuana to do that. And like all good ideas that come to you when you are stoned, they pop as if they are bubbles, off into oblivion, leaving only traces of puddles behind them.

But now I have been pot-free for more than eighteen years and I realize that it is "Ideas That Count." That is the name of the story I read while sitting at the back of my fourth-grade class when I lived at Saint Mary's Orphanage back in 1956. It is the story of how an idea brought about the first ice cream cone. I liked that story so much; I decided right then and there that I would become a writer. I zealously wanted to bring enjoyment to my readers the way that writer had done for me. Not having anyone to advise me on how to go about becoming a writer, I decided the best thing to do was to remember everything I experienced. I found out later that was a severe error. Some things need to be forgotten and I ended up relying on my pot habit to deliver me from my bad memories. Unfortunately, a side effect of pot is unproductiveness and confusion which is a steep price to pay for euphoria.

Not being able to face my feelings, marijuana helped me run away from them. Indeed, I spent most of my life running in one form or another until one amazing day in April of 2002.

At that time, I was fifty-three years old and had a near-death experience. Since I am diagnosed with sleep apnea and fell asleep sitting on my couch without my CPAP machine which delivers continuous pulmonary air pressure, my breath stopped, and I frantically fought against my spirit leaving my body. I tried desperately in vain to reach the telephone to call my son who was then twenty-three and had moved from home. I kept calling my son's name. Suddenly, this huge man of great presence sat beside me and showed me a vision. It was my son standing in the doorway of the living room, beaming and smiling with two children about ages nine and ten under his guidance. It was a lovely image that pierced my panic and brought me peace. Then I looked at the face of the man sitting beside me, but it was covered by a veil made of some mysterious smoky film of sorts. I heard Jesus say firmly, "The pot has got to go." He stood and took my left hand and with His right hand delivered glorious, fulfilling sensations and indescribable waves upon waves of love. I felt bathed in so much love emanating from that glorious touch of His hand. It was beyond any experience I ever had or could ever imagine. It was a love that I always yearned for. And then I woke up.

I used my well-honed capabilities of denial even to the point of smoking up the roaches I still had from my depleted pot stash. After smoking the roaches, I experienced the worst high of my life. The episode of Jesus appearing to me was real and no matter how much I tried to pretend it was not, I knew even while I was stoned that would be the last time I ever indulged in my pot habit, and it was. I knew the experience of the visitation of Jesus was true and I was ashamed that my Jesus had come to me not to tell me, "Well done, my child," but to tell me, "The pot has got to go."

Now, I had a new resolve and repented in remorse. My remorse was very deep. The Spirit of the Lord led me to Psalm 41:3 which popped off the page and I read: "*The Lord will strengthen him upon the bed of languishing; thou will make all his bed in his sickness.*" I marveled at the mercy of the Lord as I understood Him to point out that I had been on my sickbed for all the years I was in rebellion; I had been a backsliding Christian for a period of about twenty years. I have never been the same since that magnificent encounter with my Lord. Soon after this incredible experience, I rededicated my life to Jesus.

I trust the stories in this book bring enjoyment, hope, and even healing to those who read them. All my stories except one are in the first person. That story occurred during a period of time that I had to distance myself from. I relate this story in the third person as if it were fiction because the emotional pain is still being healed. I have experienced so much emotional and spiritual healing and often recall that wonderful day when Jesus touched my hand. One touch with His holy hand gave me new hope to press on and allow the precious blood of Jesus to clean up the pollution in my soul. Through His grace and love, I learned to forgive those who offended me and to even forgive myself for my own sins and shortcomings. God in His mercy gave me a new beginning. He gives a promise of a new eternal life that is available to all who accept the atoning sacrifice of Jesus and believe He is the Son of God who died and was resurrected to save us.

DADDY'S NOT HOME

I first remember my daddy carrying me on his shoulders on the way home from the hospital. I had been in South Boston's Blackstone Park. It must have been 1951. I was three years old. My older brothers Jerry and Lenny had been watching me in the park and I got it in my head to take off my shoes and socks and wade in the water fountain. All the adults around started to make noises that I should not do that and beckoned me to get out of the water fountain. But I was of a contrary nature and continued wading in the fountain until, sure enough, I cut my toes badly on broken liquor bottles. Next, I remember being in the hospital and feeling very overwhelmed by the unfamiliarity. Then on the way home, I bounced merrily on my daddy's shoulders as he brought me back home from the hospital.

The other early memory I have of my daddy is of a set of blocks he gave me. I remember gleefully playing with them as the sun beamed in.

My mother told me the following story when I was visiting her. My oldest brother Jerry, then about twelve years old, wanted to take me to church. My mother thought that at age three I would not behave and tried to talk him out of the idea, but he insisted that I would act right. Outside of the Catholic cathedral, my brother drew me aside. He said, "Look, we are going into God's house and in God's house no one talks. So be quiet because no one talks in God's house." Seemingly, I understood the message and sat in the pew with my hands folded politely.

Then the priest got up, went up to the pulpit, and started reading the missal for the Mass. "Now in that day," he began… whereupon I jumped up on the pew and started screaming,

"Stop it, stop it, you are not supposed to talk in church." I screamed this repeatedly even as the nuns ushered my brother and me out of the church.

I was visiting my mother because the legal authorities had decreed that my parents were unfit. They had separated me from my brothers and parents and placed me in a series of foster homes. My brother Lenny later told me that my father stopped drinking for the first three years after I was born. Then, he hit the bars with my mother following him for fear of losing her husband. They left us children to fend for ourselves and find our own food. My brother Lenny told me how he and Jerry would go into a store, plop me on the counter, and distract the store owner using my four-year-old cuteness as a decoy while one of them stole cartons of cigarettes so they could sell them to buy food to feed me and my younger brother Jimmy. I think we ate a lot of donuts. There were five us between the ages of two and twelve. Then the authorities stepped in and separated us.

From my point of view, I remembered one day sitting in a pile of building blocks while the sun streamed in the window. The next thing I knew, my entire family had disappeared. It was not until two planes crashed into the World Trade Center that I had a metaphor for what it feels like to lose everyone you love in one fell swoop. I very much identified with the children who had lost their parents on 9/11.

On the first day the Commonwealth of Massachusetts brought me to Mrs. Mahoney's house, I remember being in a room with my younger brother Jimmy. I was tossing him his baby bottle. He is two years younger than me. Then I had to go to the bathroom, and I went to a gate that was across our bedroom and called someone to help me get out so that I could go. A very cross woman came and opened the gate. I thought it was very unusual that she would be so severe with me. I pondered this puzzle while I did my duty, and the next day I was out of there.

Many years later, my "real" mother filled in the details. It seemed I had been playing in the yard when

Mrs. Mahoney started calling "Irene, Irene." Well, I just kept on playing because no one I knew ever called me by that name. All my friends and family called me "Renie." She stood over me and scolded, "Look, when your mother calls you, you answer."

I looked her square in the eye and said, "You are not my mother; my mother is big and fat and you're a skinny pickle." I then proceeded to kick her black and blue. Well, that explains why the next day I was off to another foster home and how I lost my baby brother through that separation.

Next, I remember arriving at Miss Jane's house: my new foster home. I remember that the two social workers would not let me sit in the front seat of the car and they did not seem to be very concerned about the temper tantrum I threw on the floor of the back seat. I wanted to sit in the front seat, and they wouldn't let me. Exasperated, I fell asleep and was happy to be out of their company when we arrived at my next new home. Miss Jane stood on the stoop of the side door porch, her arms akimbo. She looked OK to me.

I lived with Miss Jane for three years. She was a stout, retired English spinster who lived in a two-family house on a dead-end street in Fall River, Massachusetts. I remember my foster mother hanging out the window, voicing her perplexity from trying to understand why I was crying loudly while I ran down the street we lived on, "Yenny, Yenny." She could not figure out that I was crying for my older brother Lenny.

Coal would tumble into the chute, and me and my foster brother Tony and foster sister Linda would watch as it chunked down the shaft. There were many things to watch.

Stop and have tea with us by the path to the woods at the top of the dusty road. One small acorn is a cup and the cap is the saucer. The little grains inside brew pretend tea. Imagine! An oak tree comes from this acorn. We cavort with milkweed pods, burst them open, and spew the seeds upon the breeze. We smash open peach stones with rocks and pucker up as we taste the tart sliver of peach pit inside. We open the long green pods from the maple trees and put them on our noses.

Here comes the iceman with his ice truck. We gaze, enthralled, as he grasps ice with his long, metal tongs to deliver ice to the neighborhood housewives for their iceboxes. We leave the top of Vernon Street, which leads to the woods, and run to Main Street.

The Rag Man calls out to the ladies. He is driving a horse-drawn cart yelling, "Rags, rags!" He gets little response, but his cart is full. And we think what fun it must be to drive a horse-drawn cart!

As we venture down Main Street, we press our noses to the window and watch the Gypsy girls make bright yellow, orange, and red crepe paper flowers in their storefront. What would it be like to be in there with them twisting flowers onto pipe cleaners?

We stop by the Mobile Gas Station and romp on the old rubber tires and collect discarded Coke bottles to turn them in for their two-cent deposit. We buy licorice and Necco Wafers from the cart of the lollipop man who visits Main Street. Oh, but I see you want to go back to the woods. But not before we dawdle in front of the potato chip factory watching the miraculous production of potato chips through huge plate glass windows.

As we enter our street, the scent of lilac trees intoxicates us, and we touch and peel pieces of white bark from the birch trees. Laughing at the crunch of branches underfoot, we grab a stalk of rhubarb and wrinkle our noses in pleasure at the tangy, tart taste. I am full but there are crab apples; they are there by the path that leads to the woods. Come, walk the path and enjoy our secret place, carpeted by damp moss and enveloping us with bending trees. Let us sing our heads off here and roll about then go to the boulder with tar spilled on it and take turns sliding.

We have just enough time to pick cat-o-nine tails by the pond and pet pussy willows. Now, the sharp thistles gently pinch the skin on our fingers as we create thistle baskets with thistle handles. Not to worry; if you pet the toad's belly, you will not really get warts!

Shortly after I moved in with Miss Jane, my foster brother Tony and me were playing in the sunroom. We were both four. The radio played the song, "She's a Coming Through the Rye." I was a silly kid, and when I heard the words, "If a body meets a body," I thought it would be a good idea to pull my pants down and have Tony do the same.

There we were: walking backwards and giggling so our "bodies could meet" cheek to cheek. Miss Jane appeared at the door looking very tense, her arms folded across her chest. She yanked me up by my arms, carried me past the coal burning kitchen stove, and grabbed the steaming kettle with a free hand. She plugged the bathroom sink and filled the basin with scalding hot water from the kettle. Next, she plopped my naked bum in the scalding water. I yelled in pain and agony. When I saw Tony and realized that he was not going to get the same punishment, that left me livid with rage. In that moment of excruciating pain, I clearly realized that because Tony was favored as a boy, he would escape punishment.

This set up confusion in my mind because with my family of origin, I had been favored for being a girl. In fact, I was the first girl born after three boys. My mother later told me that she thought she could not have a girl because she had an ovary removed in a car accident. Of course, anyone with knowledge of medicine knows that the father is the one who determines the sex of the child. But my mother didn't know that and she and everyone else in the family thought that I being born a girl was a miracle. My mom told me later that I was born in a rare birth called *placenta previa* where the afterbirth arrives before the baby. In the year I was born, 1948, for a placenta previa birth, either the mother died or the baby; however, in our unusual case, both of us lived.

For the most part, I appeared to be a normal child. I mixed dogwood berries into mud and ate the "soup." It kept me home from school with a terrible rash. Looking back, I see that nature was a healing factor in the abandonment I received from my parents.

Miss Jane took us to the Catholic church, and she sent us to Catholic kindergarten and grammar school. She was a stout, frumpy lady who told us she had once been a nurse in England during World War II. I would hate it when she would clean a spot on my face with spittle on her handkerchief. She had a penchant for entering contests, and one day she entered me into the "Little Miss Sunbeam" look-a-like contest. Banana curls were planted on top of my head with an electric curling iron, and I remember being the center of attention. I did win second prize from the bread company for looking like Little Miss Sunbeam. The prize was a toy baby carriage. Since I had no doll, we used it to transport a broken wind-up clock that we liked to play with. We ran with glee while playing with the doll carriage.

When I was five, I would stare in the mirror and wonder if I had a funny-shaped head like Betsy McCall, a paper doll appearing in 1953 in *McCall's* magazine. A real treat was when we got the page to cut out the paper doll. We usually drew our own paper dolls. Even so, we did have fun. We drew a tub, cut a line where the bath water would be, and stuck the hand-drawn doll with her round bloomers and tee shirt through it. We knew we were lucky to have food; store-bought toys were for "real" children. Foster children could not expect what other children had. We just knew that.

I would wonder if my head was kind of cone-shaped because my peers in school shunned me. I did not understand it then, but I realize now there is a pecking order in kindergarten. No one who is different is accepted. I did not even know I was different. I did not know that I lagged in social development. I did not understand that my clothes were not as good as the other children's until they told me about it years later. At age five, I knew nothing!

So, there I would be, reassuring myself that the shape of my head looked all right, and I picked up the hairbrush and got it all tangled up in my hair. What a mess.

One day while coming out of the clearing of the woods, I went into the garage that was rented to a neighbor. He was a vile man who sexually abused me and gave me a nickel. Gagging and reeling from the revulsion I felt from his offense, I ran to catch up to my foster brother and sister who were lolling about the candy cart. I did not tell anyone what happened because I was sure I would get scalded again. The candy cart man sold me five lollipops tied with a ribbon and I gave him my ill-gotten nickel. When his back was turned, I stole another group of five tied lollipops because in my anger I knew that what I had endured was worth much more than just five lollipops. For the moment, I was the star who mysteriously obtained lollipops for all of us, but I felt deeply ashamed and baffled.

In kindergarten, I had a very strange nun as a teacher. I went to school one day wearing a coat that the government had sent me. It was meant to last a couple of years and was too big and felt uncomfortable, but it was a pretty coat with colored stripes. I remember the nun standing over my crayon artwork. She looked at my work, picked it up, and tore it in many pieces which she threw around the classroom. Then she made me crawl all over the classroom floor to pick up the pieces. She sent me to the corner and scolded me, saying, "You don't deserve that pretty coat you wore today." I stood in the corner in utter confusion; I did not even like the coat that was too big for me. I did not understand what had happened. Could my artwork be that bad?

My "real" mother came to visit me when I was six. I was very embarrassed and wanted to hide under the table. I had bragged to my foster brother and sister about how my mother and father were famous movie stars, which would explain why they were too busy to take care of me. I fed my fantasy by believing that songs like, "Beautiful

Blue Eyes" and "Happy Trails to You" were being sung by them on the radio just to me. Now the truth was sitting at the kitchen table: a short, fat lady with a dirty cast on her arm who claimed to be my mother. I was mortified as Tony and Linda giggled near the doorway because the fantasies I had shared with them were annihilated.

A few years later, I went to an orphanage after giving Miss Jane a very difficult time with manipulative temper tantrums. I read in the comics how "Little Orphan Annie" found Daddy Warbucks, and I begged to go to the orphanage which sounded much more interesting than living with Miss Jane. I still held resentment against her for the time she scalded me. The authorities obliged my wish and sent me to the orphanage. By then, I was eight.

St. Mary's Orphanage was in New Bedford, Massachusetts. Eighty children vied for a half-dozen nuns' attention. Newcomers were not very welcomed, which was obvious to me after several beatings in the stairwells by the other children. This went on until an older popular girl took me under her wing to protect me. Theresa had a sister my age who was half my size because I was tall for my age. She also had a brother a year younger than me. Realizing that I needed protection from the bullies, she used her popular status to save me from them.

There were people who volunteered to entertain the orphans. We had magicians and jugglers visit us. The Jewish ladies would come and talk to each of us and end the evening singing with us in a circle. My lady asked me what I wanted for Christmas and I told her I wanted a Betsy Wetsy Doll. When the gifts arrived, I was given a stick doll and was disappointed but accepted it with resignation. However, when the lady visited me again, I thanked her for the doll even though it was not the doll I had asked for. When I showed her the doll I got, she became genuinely concerned. Whoever opened the present she gave me had taken my doll. She searched the toy room, found the doll she had bought me, and made sure that I got the doll back that I asked for. I was extremely impressed that I mattered enough for her to do that.

At Christmas, they brought all of us orphans to the airport and Santa arrived in a helicopter bringing a present for each of us. So, there were good people who cared, and I believe that it meant very much to me to know that there are caring people in the world.

I stayed in the orphanage until I was ten when I found a home with a foster family.

PRETEND YOU ARE ASLEEP

In the 1950s, the ladies all hung their laundry out to dry on clotheslines. No one hung out dirty linen. Everything was brighter than bright. The most important thing was that your neighbors knew you had clean laundry in your house. Laundry was that important. This was a time when lace curtains were starched and stretched on curtain stretchers and hung on crystal-clean windows. Being clean was the only meaning. Looking good to your neighbors was the be-all and end-all.

Or, so it appeared to Renie. Renie was often stuck with the task of hanging the clean laundry from the bathroom window to the clothesline joined to a tree. The laundry always smelled fresher than fresh and was treated with bluing to make it whiter than white. The competition to appear normal and clean to one's neighbors creaked in the air along with the clothesline as it took up more clothes from the wicker laundry basket. Renie was resentful but did not allow herself to acknowledge it. Her chores seemed to be never-ending. But she did not want to seem ungrateful; after all, this family gave her a home which she had longed for at the orphanage.

She knew she would also be stuck with the ironing. In those days, everything was ironed from bed sheets to her foster father's boxer shorts. Renie also had to do the dishes all the time. She spent Saturday mornings cleaning the bathroom and dusting and vacuuming the living room and parlor. It was difficult for Renie to hide her resentment from herself. The resentment surfaced in the form of frequent daydreaming and dawdling. It was hard for her to admit consciously that she was being used, but of course she knew it on a gut level. She just could not put her feelings into words. She had attempted to protest but the comeback was an outright, "Well, if you are unhappy you can always go back to the orphanage." The two years that Renie had spent in St. Mary's Orphanage was enough to frighten her into submission.

One day when dusting, she bumped the elephant ridden by the native African warriors with their spears and an ugly crack appeared. When her foster mom saw it, she went into a tirade screaming at Renie.

Renie daydreamed about the kind of parent she would be. She swore she would never become an adult or anything like the adults around her. She would never treat a child as she was treated. In her heart, she knew if she were a "real" child instead of a foster child that her life would be a lot different. But she was clever enough to realize that she could not indulge in envy because she knew there would be no end to it. Renie learned at an early age that acquiescing to the authorities was a good way to survive. The vision that gave her the impetus to survive was her enthusiastically running to greet her future husband with a brood of children while she juggled a writing career. She loved to read and looked forward to becoming a writer. She tried to remember everything that happened to use in her future writing.

The kids in the neighborhood acted as if Renie were from another planet. It was not that Renie was ugly or stupid; she was just odd and awkward. She had landed in a neighborhood where everyone knew everyone except her. She was a too-tall, skinny young girl who, though she didn't realize it, was extremely young for her age. Nothing Renie could do was right. She was a clumsy child who never fit in, yet academically she was quick and bright. This further blighted her popularity. As a girl, she just raised her hand with the right answer a little too often. No one wanted to be her friend. She was a big baby in a too-big girl's body.

Renie was playing in Lucy's yard. Everyone liked Lucy. "Get out of my yard," Lucy demanded of Renie. Renie got angry. She was just there to make friends. A rowboat in the yard had collected rainwater. Near the boat was a pail. Renie quickly picked up the pail and dipped it in the boat to fill it with water, and then she dumped the water on Lucy's head. Lucy laughed at the audacity of this strange girl. After that, the two girls became very good friends. Lucy taught Renie to ride a bike and gave her a bike that she had outgrown. The bike was too small, but she was grateful to have a bike at all.

Renie was playing with her foster father in the living room on the couch. They were alone in the house while his wife went out one evening. He was tickling her. Renie was happy to have all this attention.

"OK," said Bill, Renie's foster father, "It's time for bed." Renie obliged. The idea popped into her head as she lay in her bed to pretend she was asleep by making loud snoring noises. Her foster father entered the room and started sexually playing with Renie. This was so shocking that she continued to pretend she was asleep. The sex games continued for the next three years.

Many nights, Renie cried uncontrollably. She learned that if she put a pillow over her head and acted as if she were suffocating herself to death that the nameless, wordless anxiety she felt would stop on the relief of removing the pillow from her face. For the most part, no one would guess the turmoil going on inside of the little girl merrily chomping down Cheerios the next morning before school. Renie psychologically learned to dissociate from herself and the sexual molestation. She had better keep her mouth shut or she would be homeless. In fact, Renie did not have the capacity or the vocabulary to say what was happening. She felt a profound unease. The stakes were way too high to talk.

There were nights she cried herself to sleep with the thoughts that nobody wanted her. Then there were nights when she said her prayers and thanked God for each and every one of her toes.

Renie prepared for the Holy Ghost Festival that would begin from their house. Pretty bouquets of artificial flowers decorated the apartment. Statues of the Madonna and other Catholic icons led the parade. Renie dressed in the proper attire: crinoline, lace, and patent leather shoes. The parade gathered and it appeared that everyone was convinced of his or her worthiness. Generally, all of those for whom they kept up appearances confirmed their goodness. The hypocrisy of it all stymied Renie.

Renie was very disturbed and only aware of the extreme alarm that she felt in her being over the molestation. She knew if she told her foster mother, she would break the family up. The conflict was that she could not allow that to happen to the very family who had rescued her from the orphanage. She did not want to break up her foster family to become like her own broken family. She continued to pretend she was asleep or to act submissive when awake and continued to disassociate herself from her feelings of fear and horror and from herself. She felt everything was all her fault, but she could not think about it.

One Halloween, when Renie was twelve, she went out Trick or Treating. That night, her foster father came into the room to remove her bag of candy. "No," Renie threatened, "if you take my candy away from me, I will tell Mommy what you have been doing." He left the bag of candy in Renie's room and never approached her sexually again.

At age thirteen she was moved to a new foster home because it was not convenient for her to be in the home that had taken her from the orphanage. In her new home, she cried frequently because she felt unloved. Her new foster mother added up the expenses she spent on her for food and clothing and realized that Renie was not cost-effective. After a few months, the Division of Child Guardianship of the Commonwealth of Massachusetts had her moved to a different foster home in the same town where she could still attend eighth grade at the local Catholic grammar school.

In her next foster home, she did not feel like calling her new foster mother "Mom." So, she did not call her anything at all. When Christmastime came, she decided to give in and call her new foster mother "Mom." Her foster mother treated this news with annoyance. Her foster father would give Renie lessons on French kissing and then give her a few bucks. She was proud to have the money to give to the missions at school. Every Sunday, the family would go to Mass, and during Lent, they would all say the Rosary in the living room together on their knees. She stopped crying from loneliness but had terrible nightmares. In one dream, a big black spider kept growing every time she stepped on it until it squashed its body on the walls, enveloping Renie with its grossness.

Renie's real mother came from Boston to see Renie graduate eighth grade. Her foster mother told her mother it was OK to take Renie back to Boston with her because she really did not want her around.

Renie lived with her real mother for the first part of the summer. Her mother told her that the Division of Child Guardianship was not pleased that her foster mother had sent her off without their permission. She hated living with her mother. She never knew when her mother's boyfriend would sexually molest her. Several children in the neighborhood knew of the vile man's predilections. Her younger sister and brother lived with their mother. They had been born after her other siblings were placed in various foster homes. They too were victims of molestation by this fiend who was their mother's friend.

Renie's mother was not around very much, and Renie deplored living with her mother. She was not used to the disorganization that her mother lived in. Often her mother would come home crying and drunk. All Renie could do in the heat of the summer was to try to clean the apartment and take care of her younger brother and sister. The Division of Child Guardianship sent a letter to her mother, but Renie got it first. She steamed the letter open. When she found out that she was going to summer camp for the rest of the summer, she cried tears of joy. It did not occur to her at the time that she did not have an address or a home.

She went to an evangelical camp. Renie was a Catholic and insisted on going to her own church on Sundays even though her doing that contributed to her being an outcast in the camp. As usual, she had the gift of anti-charisma.

As the summer came to an end, Renie became anxious that she did not have a foster home. She had been given a scholarship from her diocese to attend the best Catholic high school in the area. At the last minute, she learned she would be living with a family in Acushnet just a few miles from North Dartmouth where she would attend school.

The new foster home was a great big house that had nine other foster children, all boys. The food was good, but Renie could not get her own bath water. She had to take her bath after the boys because, as she was told, she menstruated. Large hot tears would roll down her cheeks as she bathed the best she could in the dirty, cold bathwater. Then there was that time when she was sent out in the cold New England November to wash windows of the large house that her foster parents owned. Resentment brewed in her as she performed the task with her fingers freezing and tears running down her cheeks.

It chagrined her that her foster aunt's child, who was only six, got to stay up until nine or ten at night while she had to go to bed at seven. Of course, the daughter got to take her bath first. Renie's chores were reasonable, even though she had to do the dishes every night and she did some ironing. She was not allowed to use the refrigerator and the other foster children could not go to the refrigerator, but the child of her foster aunt could do so.

For Renie, the same old story of being ostracized happened in high school. She felt a bubble surrounding her and isolating her from all the other students. She could not reach out of it. The isolation was palpable.

She did have one part-time friend. Delores would invite Renie to spend time in her apartment while they waited for a connecting school bus. The two girls would sneak cigarettes together, but Delores made it clear that she did not want to be seen with Renie once they got to school. On one occasion, Delores went to visit Renie and the two girls sneaked cigarettes in one of the empty bedrooms, and they made the mistake of leaving the cigarette butts behind. Renie overheard her foster aunt and uncle planning to send her to a boarding school. They would not tolerate someone sneaking cigarettes in their home. She was tired of being shunted around. By now, Renie realized that her fantasy mother was not something she wanted in reality. She decided that since she was tall for her age, she could find her own way in the world. She joined the ranks of runaway teenage girls.

FIFTY-TWO PICK-UP / TRAFFICKED

For those of you who never knew or do not remember, Fifty-Two Pick-Up is the name of a joke card game. You invite someone to play, and once they agree, you take the deck of cards and throw them on the floor and now they must pick them up. It is a silly joke of course, but that is how I would describe what I did to myself when I decided to run away at the age of fourteen. I literally threw myself to the wolves and let them pick me up until I ended up at Plug's house.

Skeeter Davis' song is blaring from the radio. "*Why does the sun go on shining, why does the moon glow above, don't they know it is the end of the world, it ended when I lost your love?*" I am in Plug's house and I am wiping the soot off the molding around the shelf where the radio is playing. I am picking up on the poetry of the song. The song becomes a part of me, but for the life of me I do not know whose love it is that I lost. I am not trying to figure that out. I am trying to get the soot off the molding with a damp rag.

I have always had this habit of tuning into songs and becoming part of them or rather them becoming part of me. Plug is giving me hospitality while I am a runaway. I am fourteen years old, a beanpole; if I stand sideways, you can't see me. I am tall and plain with deep-set blue eyes. How Plug got the soot all over his living room is anyone's guess. Probably one of the poker players got drunk and careless with his cigar one night. The fire happened before I arrived at the safety of Plug's apartment. It might not look safe to the authorities, but I had a bed and a roof over my head and turning tricks when the poker players got tired of poker was just part of the deal. I got fed. Franco, one of the card players, would come over with homemade soup. He never touched me. He was an older man who bragged about his twelve kids. One of his sons would come by and give me lectures on how no man would want me by the time I was twenty. I forget his son's name, but I remember he was out on bail for manslaughter over an auto accident he had been in. He was like his dad: he would not touch me either.

The man in charge of selling me to the card players went by the name of Slick. He came to me every day wearing a white sweater that he bragged his pregnant wife would dutifully wash for him each night. Billy was his friend and one of my tricks. He tried to take care of me and even helped me get a social security card under a false name. He took me out to buy clothes with some of the proceeds from the card players. He tried to steal me away from Slick. While he had me at his relatives' house, the cops came looking for me. I hid in a closet and was not found.

I was jailbait and the guys could not keep me too long, so they sold me to one of their out-of-town card players who owned a pig farm and then pulled a Murphy on him. That is, they drove out to his pig farm, took the money he paid for me, got him out of the car, and then drove off with me and the pig farmer's money. We headed up to Charleston where I would be sold to a brothel that serviced the Navy yard. I suppose it was truly fortunate that I was found by the police in the back seat of Billy's station wagon in an uncompromising position with Slick.

Slick and I were both sent to Charles Street jail because of course I lied about my name and age. Since Slick was married, we were both arrested for adultery.

For a while I adjusted very well to Charles Street Jail. After a few weeks on the run, I welcomed the much-needed rest. I had been on the run for two months. I vindictively relished the thought that no one knew where I was. Why I thought that I was punishing people I believed did not care about me was kind of convoluted since if they didn't care, why would they be worried?

I mostly stayed in my cell reading Perry Mason mystery novels and would venture out for lunch. After lunch, the other women prisoners taught me to play bid whist. Sometimes they would process my hair in the jail's beauty salon. I liked the acceptance and attention. But after a few weeks, I got tired of jail. I knew I was a minor and did not have to stay there. I got angry with the prison matron who tried to get me to clean the bathroom. It disgusted me that the task included removing dirty, used sanitary napkins pushed under the claw foot bathtubs. I flatly refused the task and they sent me to my cell. I did grow weary at the lack of fresh air and sunlight. Finally, I admitted to the warden that I was a minor and was sent to the Youth Service Board.

In 1962, I went before the Superior Court and lied under oath. The court wanted me to confess that Slick, a married, thirty-five-year-old man, had intercourse with me, a fourteen-year-old. They wanted to convict him of statutory rape.

Why did a nice Catholic girl like me lie under oath? What is the definition of a mortal sin? A mortal sin is one that cannot be forgiven. A mortal sin is when you know it is wrong, you think about it, and you do it anyway. Yes, the nuns had taught me that lying under oath is a mortal sin, but my mind had its own reasoning. Why this fellow should be sent to jail for years when he was my friend did not make sense to me. Why should he be punished for helping me as a runaway from a foster home? After all, even though I was not sexually molested at the foster home I ran away from, I knew the truth. I had been molested repeatedly in a prior home. So, in my own head, it was not wrong to lie under oath. Slick was released from custody and I was sent back to the Division of Youth Service Board. I unsuccessfully tried to hang myself in my room. From the Youth Service Board, I was sent to the House of the Good Shepherd which rejected me, then to Lancaster where I escaped after a few months of being there.

Deep inside I carried the despair that I was never to be accepted by God again. Unconscious and unmindful to me was the deep-seated feeling that the love that I lost as I sang along to Skeeter Davis' song was the love of Jesus.

It is a fact that my juvenile record was later sealed, but I am exposing my private, hidden sin because I believe that there are others who erroneously think there is no way back to the Lord after a grievous offense against God. I believed for a long time that my sin was unpardonable. But I read in the Bible that cowards do not go to heaven and I want the courage to tell the truth. And the truth is I was taught to hide. Hide the molestation and hide the fact that I was a foster child. I was even taught by my own mother not to admit that I had a Jewish grandfather. I became exceptionally good at hiding — so good that I became mentally confused to the point of developing a psychosis. And of course, that gave me something else to hide.

The Bible asks, "*Who would hide a lamp under a bushel basket?*" [paraphrase of Matthew 5:15]. When I show my light, you may see my defects, but if in seeing my defects you somehow find healing for your own soul, then there is purpose in the pain and suffering I have been through. And, if I can be an instrument in divine healing, then I am blessed and happy with the hand I have been dealt however well or badly I played it.

My stories are a spiritual path — somewhat convoluted, often torturous, but in the end triumphant as I realize I am blessed and highly favored by the Good Lord Jesus. The untwisting of my soul has been an arduous task, like untwisting a licorice stick and having it twist back to its original twisted state all over again. However, my spirit has been born again and my mind is being renewed even as I write these stories and compile this edition which is my shattered glass sculpture made of splintered puzzle pieces.

MA KATE

Ma Kate was a God-fearing "colored woman" who was set in her ways. When I first met her in 1965, I was a runaway from Lancaster Reform School. Back then, Black Nationalism was not yet prevalent in the Roxbury area (the Ghetto) of Boston, Massachusetts. A couple of years later when Black Nationalism surfaced, she told me vehemently that she just had no "truck" with such "rabble-rousers." She had called herself "colored" for seventy years and preferred it that way. Ma, the widow of a Kentucky Colonel, had spent her working life as a nurse and other than that, I know little of her past before I met her.

Ma Kate was a very influential person in my life and the first person who I knew cared about me. During the decade that I knew her, she would repeat to me, "I don't like to get angry," and, "I just want peace."

Ma was a crab on the outside, but just a softy on the inside. She had a gruff manner, but everyone who knew her saw her kindness, which was so dominant that she could not hide it even to protect herself. When pranksters would ring her bell, she would boom out a threat that she would shoot them in the knees if they were to come on up the stairs. I never knew Ma to own a gun. The idea that Ma would do such a thing even if she did have a gun was very comical and it created a feeling of safety in me to have such a fierce protector.

It was pure coincidence that I came to know Ma Kate at all. I had been speeding on some bennies and I started a conversation with her granddaughter, Mae, who was waiting at a bus stop with me. We had both just come from job interviews at the Goodyear Rubber Factory in Watertown, Massachusetts. We had applied for no experience minimum wage positions there. They turned me down because I was too underweight to meet their insurance standards.

During the long ride back from Watertown to Roxbury, Mae delighted in my non-stop conversation and invited me to her apartment. Not being able to sit still because of the bennies I was on, I cleaned up her house very thoroughly. Mae was impressed by my cleaning. She was a young, enthusiastic married mother of three children, one a toddler.

I let Mae know I was looking for a place to stay. She offered to rent a spare room to me, and I agreed to pay her a small amount of rent and to help her with the housework in exchange for the room. Intuitively, I knew that I was in trouble with the bennies and had to get away from the ready supply available at my then current rooming situation, so I was eager to move in and was happy when her husband agreed.

In 1965, bus fare in Boston was ten cents. Apartments in the Grove Hall area rented for about $75 per month for five and six rooms, including heat. But a minimum wage job of $1.25 per hour reaped a take-home pay of about $42, and even with two people working, the economic realities for a young couple with three children were constrained. Certainly, the $20 a week I paid Mae for room and board was helpful to her and her husband,

Mae quickly found out my housekeeping abilities were not very energetic once I got off the bennies and she was frankly disappointed. I doubt she ever realized that I had been hopped up when she met me.

I met Ma while I lived with Mae. She climbed the stairs to her granddaughter's apartment and stood in the kitchen, sizing me up. Ma was a big woman, tall and sturdy-looking. She had ventured to Mae's third-floor apartment solely to meet me, a fact she let me know. She wanted to know who was living with her grandchild and great-grandchildren. She was polite and reserved toward me and I felt her having met me somehow reassured her.

During the time I lived with Mae, I became friendly with her sister, Jean. She was about eighteen and closer to my age of sixteen than her sister Mae who was about twenty-four. When the rubber factory turned me down for the job, Jean brought me to her factory job where we both stood and peeled and sectioned oranges to be canned into glass jars.

After I had been living at Mae's for a couple of months, a niece from Mae's husband's side of the family was coming up North so she told me she needed my room and that I had to leave. Mercifully, she said that her grandmother, Ma Kate, would be happy to rent me a room.

I went to Ma to get her approval for moving in, and to my surprise, I found out she was not overjoyed at the prospect of taking me in. In fact, I heard her say "No," which I refused to hear since I was desperate to have a place to live. With the help of Jean, I pleaded with her.

We both convinced Ma that it would be worthwhile to have me stay with her. I kept telling her that I would not be any trouble. "You'll see," I told Ma.

This was probably the first time I heard Ma say, "Irene, I just want peace."

My job of paring oranges lasted just a few weeks before I was fired for talking back when the floor lady reprimanded me for chit-chatting with Jean. From there I walked across the street and took a job cutting chickens from a belt riding in the air in a poultry factory. I had to say I was twenty-one to get the job. I was still only sixteen.

While working on the assembly line at the poultry factory, I severed a nerve on my left middle finger knuckle. This qualified me for workmen's compensation, which I collected under a phony name and age. After that, I took typing lessons under the Manpower Development Training Act. Again, I lied to get those free typing lessons that paid me to take them.

Throughout my stay with Ma, I paid her $20 to cover my food and board. My only obligations, aside from being in before midnight and not allowing my boyfriend in my bedroom, were to keep my room clean and tend to my personal laundry at the laundromat located in the heart of Grove Hall on Blue Hill Avenue.

Ma lived on a quiet side street off the Grove Hall area of Roxbury, a place which exploded in race riots a couple of years later. Aside from the many relatives and friends who visited her, she kept pretty much to her home and was almost reclusive. I enjoyed all of Ma's relatives, especially her great-grandchildren and grandnephews.

The Grove Hall area was filled with modest, neat homes. Some tenement buildings were interspersed between the little houses. Blue Hill Avenue, the center of Grove Hall, had many stores for food, clothes, and hardware. As a young white girl living in a black community, I never encountered any difficulty until a few years later when racial tensions erupted. There were a few churches in the area that served the families of the community. Live jazz and soul music pumped out of the windows of some of the homes.

When I lived with Ma, for a year and a half, much to my appreciation, she would never let me do the dishes. Ma was very independent and insisted on doing all her own housework. Her food always tasted good and was plentiful. I often wondered at the mystery of her mouthwatering, delectable concoctions. But, then again, everything Ma touched from coffee to potato salad had the spice of love mixed in.

I had a nice, clean room, with lovely mahogany furniture. Ma was renting the top floor and attic rooms of the second floor of a two-family house. She had a parlor and living room filled with plants that flourished from her care. On sunny days, light streamed through the lovely curtain creations that graced her windows.

My relationship with Ma developed gradually. I was her roomer and she was my landlady. That in itself was mercy enough, because at my young age I would not be able to rent from a public hotel and could not afford an apartment.

Something enigmatic happened to me as I grew fond of this lady who provided me with a semblance of order through her own consistency. My personal circumstances had been extremely chaotic. I had lived a tumultuous life. I was taken away from my unfit alcoholic parents as a toddler. I suffered indignities and abuse as a ward of the State of Massachusetts up to the time I ran away from a foster home at age fourteen. I was apprehended and sentenced to a state reform school. After escaping from there, I lived with a series of acquaintances in the Roxbury area. But under Ma's daily concern, my tumbleweed life was developing roots.

Ma would ask pointed questions of me. She had a way of asking that was not prying.

She would sit on the couch with her apron across her lap and give me a quizzical line of questioning. I felt her genuine interest.

She asked, "Does your mother know where you are at?"

I told her, "She knows that I am alive."

"Where does your mother live?" Ma queried at another time.

I told her, "At the edge of Roxbury."

"Does she have a telephone?" she asked, her eyes squinting.

"Yes."

She said, "Well, I'm a mother and I happen to know that your mother would like very much to see how you are living."

Then on another day, "Irene, I was thinking it would be a good idea for you to invite your mother to dinner."

As it was, I knew social workers were breathing down my mother's neck to disclose my whereabouts. My mother was a welfare recipient, and since I was a runaway, she could not in any way endanger herself and my younger brother and sister by giving me shelter. I did know her telephone number. Even though I had not previously disclosed where I had been staying to my mother, I was able to convince her to come to dinner.

The dinner went fine, Ma being very gracious to my mother whose appreciation was apparent. When my mother left, Ma Kate took the time to tell me in a gentle but firm manner that, "No matter what, you must always respect your mother."

For her birthday, I bought Ma a parakeet. Never have I personally experienced the true joy of giving as I did that particular present. She was so tickled. Ma and the parakeet bonded immediately and every time I was around, Ma beamed her approval and appreciation to me and then nodded at the bird. There was much between Ma and me that went unspoken but rather was a relaying of feelings. Ma was like a furnace. She radiated warmth, concern, and care.

I kept my promise to be in by midnight and noticed that before Ma went to bed, she always placed a glass of water on her bedstand dressed with doilies. She studied her Bible every night. "God bless you," she would tell me and kiss me on my cheek, and I would kiss her back. One time, Ma sent away a dollar with a coupon that advertised the "Road to Life." They sent her a letter with a little tin cross inside. I sat next to Ma on the couch, watching her hold the cross vertically between her finger and thumb. She had a little smile of contentment on her face, and at that moment I glimpsed the peace that Ma cherished so much. It was intriguing.

I had a mushy side and when I would kiss Ma on the cheek, she would tell me, "Girl, if you steal all my sugar, how will I have any left for myself?" She would then look at me with a pretend mean face, mouth pursed with eyebrows touching, and I would see the twinkle in her eyes and know that it was all right to give her another hug. Then I would steal more "sugar."

But I did not keep my promise that I made to Ma of being no trouble when I begged to move in.

One time, after a lover's quarrel with my boyfriend who was later to become my first husband, I became very anxious and agitated. I ran up the flight of stairs to the roof of an overhang up in the attic of her apartment with the idea of plunging myself to my death.

Ma followed and grabbed me by the shoulders, shaking me firmly. "Don't you ever even think about doing such a thing," she sputtered with such intensity that it shocked me out of my despair. I was so bewildered by the firmness of her command that I followed her meekly down the flight of stairs back to the main apartment. We sat on the couch together and Ma glowered at me. It was outlandish to me that someone could command me not to commit suicide. It was enough to alter my mood.

Another time, I came in bragging about some clothing I had shoplifted. Ma's eyebrows shot up and we argued about my doing that. I liked the excitement and the perverse sense of getting away with something when I shoplifted. I did not know it then, but I was acting out a rage I hadn't yet admitted to myself. Ma grumbled her discontent about my bringing stolen goods to her home. "I just don't like that," she said. "It just is not right to steal."

I argued back: "If I go into a store one day when they sell an item at one price and the next day the price is slashed in half, well that means the store stole from all the people who paid full price. How can I be stealing if I am taking from thieves?"

Ma would get frustrated trying to tear holes in my argument, and she would gruffly say, "It just is not **right** to steal." But Ma never threatened to put me out.

One day, $10 was missing from my wallet. In those days, I always knew exactly how much cash I had. I had not been out of Ma's house since I had last counted my money and I didn't take it, and I was pretty sure the parakeet didn't, so that left Ma as the only suspect.

In my consternation, I just blurted out my accusation to Ma. She told me straight out, "I did not steal your money."

"Well then," I countered, ashamed even then that I actually badgered her, "Since it is only me and you in the house, how do you explain that my $10 is missing from my wallet?"

Ma moved about the room hesitatingly. I saw her hands trembling, and a look of held-back tears filled her eyes. She reached deliberately for her King James Bible and turned to the Book of Proverbs. There in the binder of the page was my $10. "I didn't steal it," Ma insisted as she handed the bill back to me with shaking hands.

I took my $10 bill with a feeling of utter confusion. How could she be telling me she did not steal it when only she could have put it in the Bible? But Ma's obvious distress overrode my incredulity. I was alarmed to see that I had upset her in this way. I had never seen her tremble and hold her body with such tension except for the time I tried to jump off her roof. Tears sneaked from her eyes. I did not know what to make of the situation. I did not know how to rest the scene in my mind. So, the scene tumbled about with no place to settle for a long time.

From a more mature view, I see Ma's discernment. It meant everything to Ma for me to know that she had not stolen from me. She took my money to give me empathy for what being stolen from felt like. She put the money in the Bible to clarify her message, "It is just not **right** to steal."

I felt sorry I had put Ma through this, and although the lesson was somewhat muddled in my very mixed-up mind, after this I was not about to bring any shoplifted items into Ma's home again. And, I did sit down and read Proverbs, which speak to me to this day. *"The fear of the Lord is the beginning of all Wisdom: and the knowledge of the holy is understanding"* [Proverbs 9:10].

Ma set me toward a path of spiritual and emotional growth. She planted a seed of faith through her love. Like her flourishing plants, she pinched me back a bit so I too could thrive. I was able to find help in a time of trouble and need.

MY MOTHER MY MUDDLE

A couple of years ago, I visited a lady psychiatrist who gave me forty-five minutes to speak of my history so she could evaluate the medication I take. At the end of the conversation, she simply said, "You had no parents." I felt a lump in my throat and fought back tears. I certainly did not want to feel sorry for myself and I wasn't sure I agreed with her. Not having parents! The best thing about having no parents would be that the Lord promised to watch over widows and orphans. In a way I am both, and the Lord has watched over me. I am not really a widow, but I might have been. If my second husband had not gone away, I might have killed him! It is a terrible thing to think you were born without parents. I have seen people who were born without arms and legs, blind, and deaf, but mostly they had parents. I had parents, but the Commonwealth of Massachusetts declared them unfit. Unfit.

When I was seventeen, I lived with Junior who would later be my first husband. We had to wait until I was eighteen to marry. During that time, Junior worked nights and I had a lot of alone time. I worked days. I had a job in a pharmaceutical company that had computers requiring me to put in the data cards. The year was 1965 and the computers filled the storehouse. Every time I would go near the computers, they would crash. I only kept the job a week and a half and they had to let me go. I guess the computers did not like my energy! So, I found another job in an insurance company but that lasted only a short time until they gave me the heave-ho.

I suspect that the insurance company got wind of the fact that I got caught shoplifting. I do not know; maybe they just didn't like my performance. They did not tell me why they fired me, so I left not knowing why I had been rejected. I had been going out on my lunch hour into Filene's and Jordan Marsh department stores in Boston proper and stealing clothes for myself. I got caught and sent to jail overnight and then to court for sentencing.

There I was: a runaway from Lancaster Reform School. I panicked. I knew I had brought this on myself, but I was very distraught. Before the judge came into the courtroom I wailed loudly and cried my heart out because I was so frightened that I would get sent to a woman's prison. If I they sent me back to Lancaster Reform School,

I would be hailed a hero because I had managed to stay on the run for over two years. I was so close to turning eighteen that woman's prison was a very real threat, and I knew it.

The judge came to the bench, read my case, and being moved by my loud crying, which I am sure he heard before he entered the courtroom, he decided, "By the mercy of the court I release you on probation for one year and you are to go live with your mother." She had shown up in court. He also added, "You will be assigned a probation officer and if you stay out of trouble for that year, your entire juvenile record will be erased." I was so relieved.

I moved in with my mother. Junior would still visit me, but I was not that happy with the situation. My mother could never live up to the fantasy mother I had longed for during my childhood, and the reality of her disgusted me. She was a short, round woman with a thick head of curly dark hair and beautiful blue eyes. She was a gad-about. She loved visiting her friends who would feed her and my younger brother and sister for the favor of her company as she gave them card readings that they all swore were accurate.

She really did have a sixth sense which she proved to me one day as I sat in a recliner near her daybed where she crocheted. I thought terribly negative thoughts about her. Suddenly, she jumped up and started punching me after having picked up on those thoughts!

I didn't like my mother and only learned to forgive her after I realized how very frightened she must have been to do some of the things she did. It was difficult to learn to forgive her, and I could only learn to do so much later in life with God's help. The other person that I had a hard time forgiving was me. But we all know by now that un-forgiveness poisons our spirit.

After the State took me away from my mother when I was four, I next saw her when I was six. While at the orphanage a couple of years later, she wrote to me and I wrote back. When I moved to my new foster home, she would write me there too and tell me her problems, such as how my brother Lenny threw a table at her. She did come to visit me for my confirmation when I was twelve and then for my eighth-grade graduation. Intermittently, from the ages of ten through fourteen, the State would have a social worker bring me to my mother's house for visits during school breaks and I would see my younger brother and sister who were born after the State took her other five children away. She would take me to the foster home of my two brothers: Freddy, who is five years older than me, and Jimmy, who is two years younger. They lived in the same foster home nearby to where she lived. I would also see my oldest brother Jerry who had recently married. Sometimes I would see my brother Lenny, who was home with her from military service.

One of the few things I liked about my mother was that aside from badmouthing my father, I never heard her badmouth anyone else. Also, she was a loving grandmother and generally loved babies. I suppose she just did not know what to do with them once they were no longer babies as she was a big baby herself. And then she told me wonderful stories of my childhood which I would never have known.

She told me about how I was born placenta previa and how I contracted diphtheria at age six months and gave it to her. She told me that they could not find me in the hospital and then they found me in the arms of a doctor who was rocking me lovingly. She told me how I was thrown out of a window at age one because of a fire, and thankfully I landed in the fireman's net. She told me that the neighbors would come to her, alarmed, saying, "Your daughter is on the roof again with her clothes off." As a toddler, I liked to pull my clothes off! She told me how when I was only three, people would come to her with their five- and six-year-olds in tow and complain because I had beaten them up defending my older brothers. She gave me an idea of my identity.

My mother was not a well woman. She had had no less than thirteen major operations. She had a rheumatic heart when she was five. Her grandmother brought her up, doted on her in her illness, and left her unable to do anything for herself.

So, the psychiatrist was wrong: I did have parents. They just were declared unfit. For years I hated the government for taking me away from my parents. I calculated all the money spent on keeping the family separated and thought that less money could have very well been spent on rehabilitating the family and keeping us together. Every time I went down that thought path, I could feel some of the rage I denied.

To illustrate the problem I had with my mother and the deep loathing I felt for her, I cite the following episode which occurred when the judge sent me to live with her.

Junior had come by and decided to take my brother and sister bowling. I did not go; I wanted my sister and brother to have some special bonding time with my boyfriend. At that time, my youngest brother Franky was eleven and my sister was twelve years old. Franky was identified as a special needs child and he had obvious problems.

When Junior came back with the two kids, he bragged about Franky's bowling. "Mrs. Pierce, you should have seen Franky bowling!"

I witnessed my mother tear my brother down by her loudly exclaiming, "Franky can't bowl; he's mentally disabled." Maybe I inherited some of my mother's sixth sense, because when I looked at the hurt on Franky's face, I immediately concluded that she had to keep him handicapped so that when he became eighteen, she could stay on welfare. I hated her for that. I suppose I judged her. And the way it worked out was that my mother died when Franky was seventeen. He did not fare well without our mother.

Shortly after our mother's death, Franky fell from a window; he ended up paralyzed and lived in a chronic care facility until he died at age fifty-one when he fell out of his hospital bed.

While I was living with her on the judge's order, we got in a fight one night and her pedophile man friend got in the mix. It was too much for me and I revealed the molestation that I had endured when I was as young as twelve by this fiend while visiting her. My mother got mad and threw me in a heap of empty milk bottles that were in a corner. My younger sister tells me she was cheering me on from the bedroom because he had also molested her and my brother.

Things were not going very well, and I moved back to Junior without the court's knowledge but with my mother's consent. She was glad to get rid of me. I did manage to fulfill the court's order though to stay out of trouble for the year.

I was ashamed of my mother. Ten years later, it was almost a relief when she died from mixing drinking with taking medicine when she was only fifty-six. Just before my mother's death, we talked on the telephone and I remember her telling me, "Renie, I read my own cards and I saw hospital bed after hospital bed." I got word of her death and left New York City to go to Boston for her funeral. At the time of her death, I was in a fragile state because I had just survived my fourth severe breakdown and suffered through a serious suicide attempt. But I forced myself to stay together because my younger sister was pregnant with her third child. I was more concerned with her than myself. We picked out a dress for my mother to wear in the coffin. It was a long, blue polyester dress with a ruffle around the collar and hem. It only cost fifteen dollars. My father, although long separated from my mother, found a way to pay for a decent funeral and burial.

I was amazed at the huge number of people who came to our mother's funeral. It was as if a famous dignitary had died. The people attending her funeral filled two floors of the funeral parlor. She had been a popular lady with her ability to read fortunes from the fifty-two deck.

In later years when I shared my feelings with my oldest brother Jerry, I told him that I thought my mother's funeral was the most dignified thing that had ever happened to her in her life. He looked at me with an angry scowl. It was just how I felt.

MAXIMUM GROWTH

I married Junior when I was eighteen. He was twenty-three. After we were married only a couple of months, I stood in the drugstore staring at the fatal label on the lighter fluid can. "If I lose my job," I thought, "this is how I will kill myself."

That Friday I was fired. I left work depressed and felt unworthy of associating with other people. Despite how bad I felt, I avoided buying the lighter fluid until Sunday morning.

On Saturday night, my husband and I had argued. The next morning, I woke to find that he had left the house without so much as a goodbye.

My intense feelings of rejection, loneliness, and vengeance carried me through the long walk to and from the drugstore. At home, I emptied the contents of the lighter fluid can into a glass.

I began to have qualms. I wondered if the clear liquid would burn my mouth, but I solved that problem by deciding to use a plastic straw. Then, I was worried that my dog might miss me.

While I was procrastinating, my husband returned home. He was inebriated.

"I'm going to kill myself by drinking lighter fluid," I told him.

"Good, go right ahead," he said. Then he slumped into a chair in the living room.

Chagrined, I sipped some of the fluid through the straw.

"Not bad," I thought.

Maliciously, I sat on my husband's lap to finish my concoction. He sat listlessly, ignoring my actions.

"Well, I'm through," I announced.

He grunted.

"Could I have a cigarette?" I persisted.

He handed me a cigarette; when I asked him for a light, he lit my cigarette.

I thanked him for the light, took a drag, and waited to explode. I finished my cigarette without exploding. A sense of foreboding filled my being. I thought dismally, "Didn't my husband even care that I might be dying?"

He pushed me off his lap, got up, and was puttering around the kitchen now; I ran to him, falling all over him. He flung me to the floor. I lay huddled on the kitchen floor and started to heave. Now more than ever I wanted to die; I forced the liquid to stay down my throat.

Then, in a timeless moment, I saw a vision. My young split-leaf-ivy plant appeared; slowly, it stretched out, reaching high and wide and growing to its maximum growth. It then began to curl and wither until it died and turned to dust. My mind immediately understood the meaning of the vision. The plant I owned was in another room, not visible in the kitchen where I lay. I believed the vision meant that the purpose of life was for me to reach my maximum growth and then die. I went to the bathroom, trembling, and forced up some of the poison. I phoned the local hospital for help telling my predicament to the receptionist in the emergency room. She instructed me to contact the police and have them bring me there.

After calling the police, I impatiently paced the floor. Minutes seemed like hours; so, I left the house to wait outside. The cruiser finally appeared, and I flagged it down as if it were a cab. The cops, amused by this, cracked jokes on the way to the hospital.

The huge examining room sparkled a brilliant white from the walls, ceiling, floor, and bedding. I felt conspicuously dirty. Three interns whisked me into the room.

"Are you the one who drank the lighter fluid?" asked one.

"Yes," I answered.

"Why isn't your mouth burned?" asked another intern, his brows knotted with concern.

"I drank it through a plastic straw," I said, and giggled at the silly sound of those words.

"She's pulling our leg," decided the third intern. "Let's get her out of here; she's wasting our time." As if on cue, the room filled with the malodorous smell of lighter fluid. Mortified, I felt my dungarees sop up the lighter fluid that had traveled its course.

"Oh Christ!" yelled one intern, running from the room. "Don't anybody light a match!"

I was examined, interrogated, put on a stretcher, rolled to a room, and put in a bed. A nurse came in, gave me a shot, and I fell quickly asleep. Later, I woke up feeling groggy, trying to place where I was.

My husband came into the room, his eyes wide, scared. I wanted to scream at the sight of him, but I forced myself to keep quiet.

Junior sat in the chair by my bed with his lips drawn into his mouth, his brow deeply furrowed. Staring at me with his still wide eyes, he took my hand, cradling it with both of his. Mentally, I detached my hand from my body. Except for the low moans of another patient, the room boomed with self-conscious silence.

"Renie, oh Renie," he finally said, forcing me to feel his presence by giving my hand quick squeezes. "The police came to the house to get me. I was dead asleep. I didn't know about anything that happened. Honest," he implored, his face all eyes, judging my reaction.

"You're a liar," I thought.

"Renie, I know what is bothering you. It is my working at night, leaving you alone so much. Things will change. I'll get a new job. Please Renie, believe me, I thought you were only drinking water. I never thought you were drinking poison. Please believe me?"

I nodded my assent, not believing a word he spoke. What I did believe was the raw fear that had crept into his speech.

"Was I dying?" I wondered, afraid to ask. He had left after I reassured him that I believed him.

The moans of an elderly male patient across the room diverted my attention.

"Why is there a man in the room with me?" I asked the nurse who had just come in to give me an electrocardiogram.

"You are in the Intensive Care Unit," she answered tersely while continuing to dab the cold petroleum to the points where she would attach the limp rubber strips.

I wished the nurse was not so businesslike. "She will never tell me my condition," I thought, and I was glad to see her leave.

The man across from me drew my attention again. He was shrouded by an oxygen tent and other hospital apparatus crowded his bed area. Through the tent he looked like a piece of shriveled, dried fruit. He was dying,

I knew. I shook away the thought that this was the room for dying people.

The old man's gallant struggle for his last few breaths awakened a deep sense of shame in me for my attempt to kill myself. I felt guilty too for the lighthearted way that I had acted in the emergency room. The curtness of the nurse made sense to me now.

Three days later, I left the hospital with a referral for out-patient psychiatric help. The spring air filled my lungs, and as I walked, I noticed all the new plant life around me. A generous sun spread its warm beams as if in encouragement of new life. And I mused at the well-timed vision of my split-leaf-ivy plant. I resolved to mend my ways. I too would try to reach my maximum growth.

DEEP IMPRESSIONS

When we married, the song we chose to play at our wedding was Smokey Robinson and the Miracles' "What Love has Joined Together (can't nobody take it apart)."

I met Junior when I worked with him at the laundry where we pressed uniforms. I operated the press for work shirts, and he operated the press for pants. I was being paid a penny a piece for each shirt that I would send into the shirt press. I pressed the body of the shirt and my co-worker pressed the sleeves. On a good day, I would press thirteen hundred shirts. That was thirteen dollars per day before taxes. Junior liked me and kept asking me out. But I declined only because I had a boyfriend at the time and the last thing I wanted was two men fighting over me. But I broke up with that boyfriend over his jealousy of my friend's brothers. The next time Junior asked me out to a party I accepted, and we became close. At work, I looked over at his sinewy, well-built body as he pressed pants with his own shirt taken off to bear the heat from the steam. Salt would be on his beautiful dark skin to the point where I would just want to reach over to brush it off. Junior had been a high school football player and he was handsome and built.

Since I was only sixteen when I met Junior, we had to wait until I was eighteen to marry. We were both eager to do so. Junior was a fierce protector; I genuinely loved him, and I believed he loved me. My older brother, Lenny, warned me about interracial marriages. He told me that marriage was hard enough for two people of the same race. I had a mind of my own and ignored his advice. I honestly believed that love could solve all problems as they came along. I did not know it at the time, but Junior's life was complicated by a bad memory of seeing his dad lynched by the Ku Klux Klan when he was only five years old and lived in Fayetteville, North Carolina.

The polarization of Boston where we lived was familiar to me. Boston had its hub in the business center where various ethnic groups could work and shop. Everyone knew the spokes on that hub had clear demarcations for varying cultural enclaves. I knew which sections not to go visit with my black friends. The subways were neutral. Roxbury, where we lived, before Black Nationalism, was safe for interracial couples. I knew Cambridge was safe, but the North End was not. East Boston was "iffy" in 1966 but nowadays would present no problem for interracial couples. Brookline, Brighton, Back Bay, and Beacon Hill were not economically feasible when it came to renting. South Boston was out of the question on all counts. That is just the way things were.

Our marriage was only a few months along when we separated due to our mutual immaturities. I put our furniture in storage and went back to live with Ma Kate. Junior went to live with his brother. Then he came down with reactive arthritis that landed him in the hospital. Even though we were separated, I could not abandon Junior in his crippled condition. The doctors told Junior he would never walk again. Junior, always proud of his athletic physique, was maimed by the arthritic disease at age twenty-three. His normally charismatic charm was somber, and he was withdrawn.

After Junior was discharged from the hospital, we moved into my married friend Barbara's spare bedroom. Ma Kate would not have Junior living in her home. Junior lay helpless on our bed with his legs resembling limp spaghetti strings dangling within the confines of the casts. The doctor had put the casts on with buckled straps so we could remove them and air his legs out as needed. I was resigned to Junior's crippled condition. But Junior had ideas other than to accept the doctor's diagnosis.

One night when I brought him the bedpan, he flung it from my hands. Rage bolted out from his eyes. He sat upright and unbuckled his casts. I was shocked at what happened next. Junior threw himself against the wall of the bedroom and then flung the trunk of his body from wall to wall of the corridor which ran from the bedroom to the bathroom. He threw his body against the wall, thumping his upper arms against it in such a way that his shoulders were literally banging from wall to wall while his legs dangled below him. He reached the bathroom and never allowed me to bring the bedpan again. I witnessed Junior literally willing himself to walk. After home-made physical therapy, two months' time, and attention, he was able to walk again despite the doctor's diagnosis. I viewed it as a divine healing.

In the late spring, we moved to our new rented apartment which was the first floor of a two-family home sporting a wild rose bush near the small front porch. It was a neat one-bedroom apartment located near the heart of Grove Hall in Roxbury. Junior walked but could not work and it appeared to me that the first place he walked to was to the liquor store. God only knows how much pain he was in.

When I got home from my full-time job typing address labels, I cooked dinner and headed out to my part-time job at Kemp's Hamburgers. At the time, I worked close to seventy hours a week. I worked typing address labels in the day and went to Kemp's after dinner. I aimed to pay off our furniture storage bill to get the rest of our belongings home. We had a very tight food budget.

The miracle of Junior's walking moved me so much that whenever his friends were over, I would stretch out our dinner and feed the half-dozen friends that showed up. I literally lived my own version of the "Loaves and Fishes." The clamor of good-natured jokes filled the kitchen, and Junior's charismatic smile returned. He seemed to thrive on their company.

Wayne the preacher's son stands out in my mind. He would show up but would decline to have dinner with us and sit in the living room with his cap in his lap. I believe he was praying that there would be enough food for everyone, and there always was. His cap was always with him, respectfully removed during his silent prayers, and the guys laughed about that.

Working those long hours took a toll on me. There would be times when I rang up food at the cash register at Kemp's that I had the illusion I was floating off the floor. One day at home before work, I turned on the gas in the oven and went searching for a match to light it. I underestimated how much time the gas had been on. When I lit the match and opened the oven door to light it, it seemed as if the whole kitchen swooshed with the sudden expulsion of lit gas. I quickly slammed the oven door shut; the only thing I did right. My eyebrows were singed, and I was burned on my arm and hand that had held the match. On the way to the emergency room, I joked with Junior in the back seat of the taxi saying, "Oh look, now I am a *Renie roast*." That was a silly pun on my nickname that I invented to lighten the mood. The incredibility expressed by the taxi driver put me in touch with how really not funny the incident was. At the hospital, they washed my burns with disinfectant, giving me instructions to continue using it at home, which I did. I continued with my lengthy hours working the two jobs.

During the hot summer of 1967 when the guys showed up at the house bringing us news of the ongoing race riot, the normal hubbub of jokes was missing. There were nervous and excited rumors jangling in my ears as I tried to stretch yet another meal. I heard, "The cops cracked his head open while he was sitting on his porch," and other horrifying reports. I was too busy to check with the newspapers to find out more of what was happening and did not know what started the riot in our area.

My rented apartment was located only four blocks from the shopping area where the riot occurred. The next day, which was Saturday, when I reached the shopping area the reality of the devastation was out of a nightmare. While shopping for food, the blight of debris and shattered glass stunned me. I felt puzzled and depressed about the turmoil that had struck our neighborhood. The results of mayhem were everywhere. The smell of fear and rage fouled the air. The music that ordinarily pumped out of the houses that I passed in my daily travels had stopped playing.

I was more horrified than afraid. I made feeble conversation with the hardware store owner, a Jewish neighbor. I felt sorry for the shop owners who had the enormous task of sweeping up the mess, repairing the broken glass, and running business as usual. This kind of violence did not make sense to me. It left a negative, ominous feeling in my head to walk about the area and try to get my errands done among the wreckage.

Considering the chaos in our midst, the group of our usual visitors decided to escape to Revere Beach and enjoy a cotton-candied day of rides, sea air, and the victory of winning cheap, plush animals. Revere Beach was an hour's subway ride away. About six of us went. After we had our fill of salt air and fun, we rode the subway back to Dudley Street Station in Roxbury where we found that the busses going to Grove Hall had stopped running because of the race riot. We were informed that there was an 8:00 p.m. curfew; it was past curfew. With no other means to travel home, the group of us decided to take the twenty-five-minute walk. We steered clear of the wrecked avenue.

The night was too quiet. We became vaguely uneasy and perhaps that is what inspired us to break out in the wonderful harmony to the verses of the song by The Impressions: "Amen." We sang, heading to our homes, some of us carrying stuffed animals that we had won.

Suddenly, three patrol cars swung alarmingly upon us in the night. About eight riot squad policemen jumped out of their cruisers and came at us with their riot batons. These were not billy clubs but three-foot-long riot batons. One cop came at me and smashed me with great force just above my stomach. Time stood still. Incredibly, Junior was on the ground being beaten on the legs. Horrified, I screamed at the top of my lungs, "I'm pregnant, I'm pregnant!" (I wasn't, but how would the police know that?) I screamed so loud that it drew out from the corner tavern a group of black men glowering angrily at the police who now backed off. The cop, who had rammed me in my solar plexus which I was now clutching, stopped to ask me what we were doing out there. Shaking, I told him I was walking home with my husband. With a contrite look that was skewered with shame, the cop drew away from us and headed back to his cruiser with the rest of the riot squad who withdrew back toward their cruisers.

As we walked home, Junior limped; our friends tried to lighten up the episode and joked about how when the cop had beat Wayne over the head, Wayne had tipped his hat, nodded his head, and said, "Thank you, sir." They laughed about how our friend Roger had simply kept walking in a businessman's stride as if he was not part of our group. But our laughter was laced with fear and echoed awkwardly in the evening air. Everyone went home.

Junior and I sat on our front porch. He was rubbing his legs and I was holding my mid-section. I trembled uncontrollably and I was livid with rage. I wanted to strike back at someone, anything. I wanted to run to the newspapers with my outrage at this offense. As I expressed my feelings to Junior, he talked me out of any action that I might even think of taking.

He asked, "Why should it be a white person that has to draw attention to what happened?" I looked into his eyes and saw the anguish of a man who did not want his wife to defend him. I knew he would not defend himself.

I did surreptitiously go to the Dudley Street Police Station the next day to complain. I was told, "They were just scared young white men from the suburbs."

I do not think it coincidental that a couple of months later, I had my first psychotic episode. Indeed, insanity is a viable alternative to reality.

WHEN THE MIND CALLS FOR TIME OUT

We had a terrible fight and I left Junior. I packed my bag and took a cab to a friend's house. As I rode in the cab, I could hear Junior howling like a dog even though the cab had already traveled quite a distance. I believe that is when my fragile state began deteriorating, because although the howling seemed real to me, it is unrealistic that I could have heard it from that distance. At my friend's house, chaos soon erupted there when her estranged husband barged in the house yelling while her children ran under the bed. I was shaking for them, my friend, and myself. After her husband left, I remembered I had promised to babysit for my other friend's three-year-old while she went to her night job. So, I made my way across town by taxi over to her apartment to keep my word. Her child was sleeping, and I had a few hours of peace to calm down until my friend came home around 2:00 a.m. We smoked reefer together. To this day, I do not know if it was laced with some other chemical or if my fragile state of mind revolted, but I spun into an altered state of awareness where everyone's face was dripping down, even in pictures.

When this condition persisted into the next day, I realized I needed help and made my way to Massachusetts Mental Health Center. I knew of them because I had received out-patient help after my episode of swallowing lighter fluid. After an intake interview, which appeared to me to be the judgment by angels in heaven, I was admitted to the Clinical Research Center where a special program studying schizophrenia and plasmapheresis research was being performed. I was given medication which looked like a hairy eyeball, and I was so far gone that when food was brought to me on a tray, I tried to make pictures out of it with my hands. Since I have always relished my food, it was extreme that I was unable to correctly identify food. Odd things happened.

I entered into the artwork on the walls and had visions of an amusement park that was not there out of my window. I remember hazily that I found myself on the bathroom floor talking to the dust. Then, I spent considerable time lying in my bed as I fantasized that I was taking a trip as a feather going through my mattress.

I had my first sane moment when a lady appeared over my bed dancing, smiling maniacally, and jangling a string of bells in her hand. I thought, "This lady is crazy, and I better not let her know I am afraid." So, I smiled. We became quick friends and Joan shared her time with me in the occupational therapy room while she was visiting four young children. We painted and did activities. Gradually, after a couple of months, I grew well enough to go back home. Joan and I remained friends until she died forty-eight years later. I left the hospital with Junior who had come to take me home.

I had a job typing labels in a mail order house. This work was waiting for me when I got out of the hospital. Junior had a heroin habit which kept him out of the house most of the time while I was home. I was lonely and bored and ended up leaving him after a couple of months. I went to live with my new friend from work: "Mother Earth."

My friend was very nurturing and artistic in spirit. She encouraged me to draw and paint pictures while we listened to the Beatles. We enjoyed a great friendship. Her wit and humor often surprised me and uplifted me. She did an impersonation of Eleanor Roosevelt declaring: "We must share our abundance with the world. Good luck is part of that abundance. Franklin always used Good Luck in the White House." Another time she went on her back porch and shouted the words to the Habitat Soup jingle in a terse English accent: "You mustn't, you mustn't, you positively mustn't, put water in your Habitat Soup. It's simply unbelievable, utterly inconceivable, that anyone would ever, ever stoop, to putting water in their Habitat

Soup." Well, I suppose you would have had to have been there! After a few months, I did get my own apartment a few blocks from her in East Boston. I continued my pot habit. I had quit all my medications, not believing I needed them, but then I entered another period of delusion. I remember being in a catatonic-like state believing that the whole world had been called to judgment, but I had been forgotten. During this time, I did not eat, sleep, or even go to the bathroom. I am not sure how long I was in this state, but I believe it was several days.

My friend Joan who I had met in the hospital got worried about me. She came by my apartment, saw I was not in my right mind, made me some soup that tasted weird, and got me dressed. We took the subway back to Mass. Mental Health Center. I stayed there six months. My job was held for me and I went back to Junior who had come to get me. Again, I stopped taking my medicine.

Junior was still out of work due to his disability, and he had a subsidized apartment facing Franklin Park, in the Roxbury section of Boston. He was still on heroin which I discovered when our apartment was raided and the needle works were found. But I could have guessed his habit. When I arrived at his apartment, the only food that was in the house was a box of oatmeal. When a user eats uncooked oatmeal, it swells in their stomach and makes them feel full. That leaves more of their funds for heroin. After a couple of months, I left Junior. We had a fight which netted me a black eye for winning a hand of bid whist while I was paired opposite of him. I packed a paper bag with my belongings and called my friend Joan the next day from work and she helped me get a place to stay.

My life was very chaotic at the time. I found my way through working and friends. I studied for my GED and started going to college at night. I ended up getting a year of credits earned part-time at night at Harvard University School of Extension Studies. And later, when I moved to New York City, my job paid for another year's worth of credits at New York University School of Business. I always found work and was a good worker. But, two years after my second breakdown, I ended up in the Eric Lindemann Mental Hospital when I had my third severe psychotic episode. I was in an extreme manic state; I had even signed up at a local church as a volunteer to help the elderly, homeless, and needy. I stayed at Eric Lindemann located in the center of Boston for a month and was diagnosed as Manic Depressive. I was depressed that I was unable to perform any of the volunteer work that I had signed up for. I was put on lithium which I stayed on for a couple of years until I met my son's father who easily convinced me that I did not need it.

During the late 60s, I did seek meaning through religious experiences. There were all sorts of groups around. I studied with the Jehovah's Witnesses for two years and ended up at a Hare Krishna temple in my travels. I studied Hatha yoga and meditation and learned to calm myself down. I remember once, while near

Harvard Square, someone came up to me and told me they wanted me to go with them to show me where Jesus was. I declined, because I had read in the Bible not to go with anyone who said that.

In retrospect, while struggling to keep my sanity enough to operate in the free world, I came to my own conclusions about mental illness. I believe that if there is enough psychological pain, the brain kicks in to help by spilling chemicals freezing over certain parts of it in order to cope with the bombardment that it is experiencing. That probably is an oversimplification. However, I do see the connection between the fact that when I decided to abandon my suicidal ideation, I had no outlet for the tension, anxiety, fear, and subsequent psychological pain I experienced. I do recognize that there is a genetic component to what is now called bipolar disorder, and there are others of my family members that have been affected. I would call this a genetic predisposition that can be aggravated by assaults on the senses.

When I was in Bellevue during my fourth psychotic episode, I convinced all the patients on my ward to reject their medication. This perturbed the staff so much that they told me the only way I could get out of Bellevue was to reverse my persuasive influence. Of course, I complied.

Having to deal with the reality of my illness despite my denial of it gives me both humility and compassion. I had to learn self-care. I had to learn to watch myself. I had to learn to take my medication. I can easily identify with others who have mental challenges.

I took myself off medication throughout my pregnancy and stayed off it up until the time I had another psychotic episode four years later. I nursed my son, so I knew I could not take medication then, and I erroneously believed that I just did not need medication. I had a severe breakdown when my son was four years old. When I returned to my church after that breakdown, I was told, "Go to Dr. Jesus; you don't need medication." But that was wrong advice. It is with humility that I finally learned I must take medication.

UP FROM SUICIDE

I was visiting Mother Earth, which is my nickname for my good friend of over fifty years. It was 1974 and she had moved to the lower East Side of New York City from Boston where I met her in 1968. I met her at a job we had of typing names and addresses for a mail order house. This was the job I had before my first breakdown, and my typing was fast enough to merit my job being held until I was able to return to work. I was in a shell-shocked state of mind. We sat at desks facing each other and she later admitted I was so far in a shell that it scared her. Being creative, my friend found a unique way to draw me out. She had been involved with Summer Stock Theater and knew how to throw invisible boogers. She would pull out the imaginary booger from her nose, squint one eye, and then in an exaggerated manner toss it across the desk to me. I believe God in His divine wisdom knew that her sense of humor was exactly what I needed to leave my withdrawn state.

During my visit to her in New York City, Sammy showed up at her apartment. When I met him, our eyes magnetically locked as if we each knew we had a destiny together. I was embarrassed because this was my good friend's admirer visiting her. So, I dismissed myself and went across the hall to visit Mother Earth's neighbor. Amy, confined to a wheelchair, was happy to have my company. A couple of hours later, Mother Earth came by and told me she wanted me to go to Bear Mountain with her, Sammy, and her other friend. She let me know that her friend Paul was driving us up to have a great day there. I agreed and found myself paired with Sammy in the back seat while she was paired with Paul in the front seat. Sammy was a natural-born wit and had me rolling in laughter all the way from New York City to Bear Mountain, New Jersey. He was tall, handsome, intelligent, and witty. This was a wonderful combination to me when I was twenty-six and looking for a significant other. We had a great time. I remember that as we passed Palisade Park before it was torn down, this was the vision I had seen from the hospital window during my first breakdown. Later, we were on the Hudson River in a canoe and I remember jumping off the canoe in the middle of the water, sinking to the bottom, and gleefully cranking my arms up and down until I hit the water's surface. I felt like I was reborn.

The romance was a whirlwind. Since I lived in Boston and he lived in the Village in New York City, maintaining our relationship required a few bus trips back and forth. When I was thinking something, he would give me the answer in a letter before I could ask him. I was greatly impressed. At the time, neither of us had telephones. On one of his visits he set up a chess board and blindfolded himself and played a game against me and won. Then, he took the blindfold off and went over the game move by move from memory, explaining why my moves needed improvement. I thought this man was a genius. Sammy was younger than me by five years. He had quit college because of a bout with food poisoning, and he had a job as a freight elevator operator in a loft building.

I had been upfront with Sammy about my mental illness from the beginning. Before I met him, I had three "nervous breakdowns." I was on Lithium and he told me to quit. We both agreed that if I had an episode, he would work me through it. About four months after I had moved in with him, I went into a full-blown psychotic episode and lost my secretarial job because I was acting bizarre at work.

Sammy took care of me and did not bring me to a hospital as we had previously agreed. I stayed in my psychotic state for several months and have little memory of what a nuisance I must have been. I do have a memory of sitting on the stoop to the loft building where we lived in and clucking like a hen. In fact, after several months of being in severe psychosis, I was starting to come back to reality without any medicine.

One day I ventured out and walked to the Wall Street area. I went into the Bank of America and got extremely frustrated when they refused to cash a personal check for five dollars. I did have identification but was not their customer. I started screaming at the top of my lungs, "America, America, where is America?" I was deposited in a paddy wagon and brought to Bellevue Hospital.

At the hospital, I was put into restraints and dosed up with enough psychotropics to put me in a twisted, pretzel-like state. When Sammy came to visit me, he literally had to pry my arms and legs from their contorted state. I stayed long enough (about a month) to be considered stable enough to leave. Upon my exit, the doctor asked me what medication I wanted to take. "Librium, Haldol, Valium?" he ventured.

"Valium," I thought, "that sounds so valiant." I told him I wanted to take Valium. Little did I know that Valium was a depressant.

I had been in a manic state for several months and was already in the depressed version of the disorder. I went back to the loft with Sammy. He would visit me from his job at lunchtime. I started having suicidal ideation but did not share my thoughts with him. I was so ashamed of what I had put him through with my psychotic episode and saw how futile our love relationship looked for the future. I was very depressed and wondered why I even bothered to brush my teeth. One day, after Sammy left from his lunchtime visit to go back to work several blocks away from our loft, I decided to down the whole bottle of Valium.

I dazedly remember him carrying me to the freight elevator from our fourth-floor loft apartment. Then I woke up in a wheelchair in the hospital. My first thought was, "Oh, I can't even commit suicide right, and look at me: I am in a wheelchair. I probably will never be able walk as punishment." I no sooner had that thought when a flood of victorious joy ran through my body. I knew I could walk. I stood up and found my way to the recreation room of the hospital and found a Bible. I knew intuitively that God had spared me from my attempt to kill myself and I was grateful because I did not know that God cared anything about me. For a long time, I had thought that I was beyond His mercy. I went to the hospital chapel on Sunday and my mood was so positive that Bellevue let me leave the hospital after only one week.

Sammy filled in some of the blanks for me. He had been in his office at work where he waited for the tenants who needed the freight elevator. He had a premonition that something was wrong and decided to come back to our loft several hours before his quitting time. When he found me, he carried me out onto Bleecker Street, put me in a cab, and brought me to Bellevue. They left me on a gurney in the hospital hallway and he loudly insisted that they pump my stomach. As he loomed with his imposing

6'4" frame, the staff complied. I was out cold for three days after they pumped my stomach.

The first time I tried to commit suicide, I was only ten. No one knew what I was doing. I would take a pillow and try to suffocate myself with it. Then, when I reached the point of suffocation, I would remove the pillow and immediately feel relief. This kept up for several years. During my teen years, I tried various methods of suicide. At age fifteen, I tried hanging myself while at the Youth Service Board. While I was at Lancaster Reform School, I broke glass and chewed it. When I was sixteen, I was distressed because my boyfriend (later my first husband) was in trouble with some loan sharks and he had seemingly disappeared. I went to an alley and tried to slit my wrists with a Gillette razor blade. This was the kind of blade that came out of the container one at a time. As I sat on a fire escape in the alleyway, slashing my wrist, I had no success. Then I became awestruck when I realized the reason for my lack of success was that instead of one razor coming out of the container, two had stuck together and that had blunted the blade from its efficiency. That realization, along with a nun peering through a half-shaded window across the alley, was enough to creep me out of my destructive mission and I got up and walked, dripping blood from my wrist, to the nearest Emergency Room where they dressed my wound.

Whenever I got in a tough spot, I would have suicidal ideation. But, after I swallowed a can of lighter fluid at age eighteen and ended up in the intensive care unit along with people who were fighting to save their lives, my good sense kicked in and I promised to do better and not to allow myself to give in to self-pity and self-destruction. Interestingly, a year later I started having psychotic breakdowns. In retrospect, it was as if deprived of the outlet of suicidal ideation, my mind revolted and threw me into psychosis. Truly, there were very stressful situations going on in my life even if some of them I brought on myself.

Before I met Sammy, I had three psychotic breakdowns. My diagnosis ranged from acute schizophrenia to manic depressive. Each time I had a breakdown, I was put on various psychotropics: Thorazine, Haldol, and Lithium. After release from the hospital, each time I would quit taking my medication. I didn't believe I needed it.

It is important for me to state here that my personal belief from a relative state of wellness is that to have suicidal tendencies and ideation, or to commit suicide, indicates one who is not well. Anyone who commits suicide is not in their right mind.

Having been unsuccessful in my attempts gives me the opportunity to conclude that all I ever did was try to escape the emotional pain I suffered. I realize that this might not apply to every case, but if you have lost a loved one to suicide, I hope you realize that the chemical imbalance which occurs with this great depression is not something that you or your loved one are responsible for. I do believe in the mercy and grace of God. I was taught that the sin of despair results in eternal damnation. But I do not believe a good and merciful God would do this. And I do believe that God is good. I know from experience that there is often vindictiveness in taking one's own life. The irony is that although the mood convinced me at the time that I am unloved and/or unwanted, I still thought that I could punish people who didn't care. But if they didn't care, why would they be punished? My thought is that kind of convoluted thinking really is a disease. Since I know this firsthand, I doubt very much if our merciful God would punish someone for being sick. When I say by grace I am saved, I mean it.

Problematic is the stigma attached to mental illness. I can go to a job and talk about my thyroid problem or any other physical problem, but the moment I admit to having a mental problem, I am in trouble with my job. I will not be trusted. In fact, I only feel comfortable writing this because I am now retired. With the stigma attached to mental illness, a person suffering from extreme anxiety and depression cannot seek help very easily. Of course, finding good psychiatric help is often a great challenge, but it is even more so because of the shame attached to needing help.

It is OK to ask for help when you need it. The whole ordeal of hiding mental illness is exhausting and creates an anxiety in and of itself. But, if you think about it, why is it more shameful to need help for a disorder of the mind than for any other physical ailment? After all, the brain is an organ and is just as entitled to go awry as is any other organ in the body.

I remember working with a very prominent attorney who had a client come in to visit when he was in the middle of a psychotic episode. I was startled that this intelligent, Harvard-trained attorney acted like his client's disease was something that he might catch if he were not careful. And, as I observed the attorney's body language (he was flicking off the man's essence from his clothes as if it were cooties he could catch), I was very thankful that I had never revealed to him my own malady which at that time was under control with medication. So, the stigma is real, and I admit that I spent a large part of my life pretending I was normal. I did it so long that I think in due time I actually became normal. But I still take my medicine every day because I learned the hard way that if I do not take my medication, I might spin into a psychotic episode at some point. I am normal for me!

In this life we all have our crosses to bear. My cross actually turns out to be a little cross compared to the crosses carried by other people. I only hope that somehow the mess of my life is turned into a message of hope and understanding to people who need help. I think often of the fact that when the Good Lord Jesus was climbing up Calvary hill with His cross, He needed help to carry it [See: Matthew 27:32]. I think that vision is placed in the Bible to teach us that if the Son of God needed help, it only stands to reason that we have the right to ask for help when we need it. Another vision that is important to me is the Last Supper. When Jesus washed His disciples' feet, He also washed the feet of Judas who He knew was about to betray Him [see: John 13: 1-20]. That vision humbles me. I know that I would have a hard time serving someone who was about to betray me.

It gives me a goal to head toward; to become Christ-like is a lifelong venture. I have learned that I cannot fight my devils on my own. I need Jesus to fight my battles for me. Every day is a daily battle. An important strength that I have gained from managing my psychosis is to be able to watch myself and notice when I am acting out my stressful feelings. Then, I know I must take care of myself and give myself time to recover from whatever is stressing me out. On a daily basis, to help me fight my battles I meditate on the armor of God, the Ephesians' Armor (See: Ephesians 6: 10-18), and imagine myself putting it on piece by piece to protect me that day. I spend time in thanksgiving and praise. Hey, I have been given another day to redeem the time! (See Colossians 4:5.) I spend time every day reading a portion of the Holy Bible from beginning to end with time for reflection. I read daily devotionals. It takes me about a year to read and study the entire Bible.

By beginning my day with a focus on God, I can attest that He is more than enough, and He inhabits the praises of His people! (See Psalm 22:3.) Realizing this truth gives me purpose and strength to continue to be grateful for my life, and praising God for all He has done comes easily. I can thank God for all my difficulties because He has been faithful to me even when I was oblivious to Him. Salvation is a process, and ultimately my tribulations brought me closer to Him. First comes justification, then sanctification — and that for me is an arduous process. But I have glorification to look forward to and that gives me hope. Psalm 40 verses 1-3 say it best:

I waited patiently for the LORD; and he inclined unto me and heard my cry.

² He brought me up also out of a horrible pit, out of the miry clay, and set my feet upon a rock, and established my goings.

³ And he hath put a new song in my mouth, even praise unto our God: many shall see it, and fear, and shall trust in the LORD.

AND GOD LAUGHED

It's amazing how an intelligent person can overlook the love of God for so long. My convoluted thinking made me believe that I was too much of a sinner for God to love me. In my late teens, I would gaze off longingly in the distance at churchgoers going into church and just believe that I was not good enough for God. Though I made some attempts, but I felt very deeply that I was not good enough for God.

How I missed the entire story of redemption is beyond me. Christ died to save sinners. [See: 1 John 1:9; Romans 5:8; 1 Timothy 1:8-11; 1 Timothy 1:15; 2 Corinthians 5:21; and other verses.]

I turned my life over to Christ while watching *The 700 Club* in 1977. That is when my life changed. In my late teens, I had two hospitals tell me I couldn't get pregnant without two major operations, and in my late twenties,

I was busy trying to make my mark professionally so I would be in a financial position to adopt children. Soon after I accepted Jesus as my Lord and Savior, I got pregnant.

I had been walking down Pine Street in the Wall Street area of Manhattan, going toward my secretarial job, when I spotted a pregnant woman a short distance in front of me. I felt a sensation of movement in my abdomen and a voice within me said, "Don't be jealous; I'm right here." That is how I knew I was pregnant. I was only about one month along. I stopped taking my medication to protect my unborn child. The doctor I was seeing for prenatal care would not confirm my pregnancy until he heard a heartbeat. He thought I was having a hysterical pregnancy. So, my son communicated with me while he was being formed in the womb before a heartbeat could be heard.

I was twenty-nine when I conceived. I was still in therapy, and the therapist tried to talk me into an abortion because of my mental health history. The doctor said to me, "Well, it looks like you don't have a choice."

And I asserted, "No, I have no choice; I must have this baby." She accused me of wanting to have a baby to cement a bad relationship together, but no accusation or argument could make me terminate my pregnancy. In fact, I terminated therapy which took place at Bellevue Hospital. I was afraid that they would put me in restraints and end the pregnancy for me.

It was true that I was in a bad relationship, but I ended up marrying Sammy and hoped for the best. I wanted a family very much. In fact, as I think about it now, dreams of having a family helped me survive my childhood.

Motherhood agreed with me. I spent days on end bonding with my baby. I went to the library and found books that guided me into helping him with his development. I exercised him on a beach ball. He was a good baby. We watched *Sesame Street* together, and by the time he was ten months old, he knew his alphabet. He could recite it and identify any letter as it was shown to him even out of order. I was blessed with a highly intelligent, healthy baby.

I had six months of maternity leave (only two months were paid leave, and I had taken out a loan to financially survive the other four months). When my leave was up, I had to find a babysitter. I got on my knees and prayed for one with tears streaming from my eyes. I did not know anyone in the town of West New York, New Jersey where we had moved to at the beginning of my pregnancy, and I was distressed about the fact of leaving my son with a stranger.

After I prayed, I remembered a little girl who had helped me climb the stairs to my fourth-floor apartment with my groceries. She was so polite and had flatly turned down a tip that I offered her. I thought, "She must have a very good mother." I knew the little girl lived in the building, and I believed she lived on my floor. I went to the door that I thought was hers and asked her mother to babysit for me when I went back to work. The mother turned me down. My heart was crushed but I remembered that God answers prayer when you have faith, so I went to the lady on the third floor who I had seen in the park with her son. I figured she was a good mother because at least she took her son to the park. She also turned me down but told me that Suzy next door might babysit for me. I went to Suzy and thought, "Ah, this is my answer." Suzy's husband was busy helping his two children with their homework. A picture of Jesus hung on their kitchen wall, and I thought, "This must be the babysitter God is going to give me." When I asked, they too turned me down but told me to go to the apartment below them on the second floor and ask Maria. Maria came to the door with a big smile. She agreed to babysit for me. Oh, by the way, it turned out Maria was the mother of the polite little girl who helped me with my groceries.

Maria's family was so good to my son; the whole family, which was comprised of three children and her husband, not only cared for my son but loved him. We are friends to this day over forty years later. So, when I prayed for a babysitter, I not only got one, but I also got a friend and family that has stood by my side through thick and thin throughout the years. Not only her nuclear family stood by me but also her extended family became part of our lives. After I had been going to Maria's house for about a year, I remarked to her one day that no matter what problem she had, she always had a smile. She told me, "That's because I always pray to Jesus every night." Then the light dawned in my spirit. I realized this friend that I had prayed into my life led me to a closer relationship with the Lord just by being a kind, loving person. She brought me closer to learning to trust in the Lord. She was a walking Epistle.

When my son was about sixteen months old, at a chance encounter at the bus stop a very outgoing young lady invited me to her church and told me a van would take me and my son to her church. I started going to West New York Assembly, a Pentecostal church, which at the time was very much geared toward children. All the songs were sung with hand movements as if for the deaf. I relish to this day the memory of my son walking down the aisle to the altar and putting pennies in the steeple of a replica of the church for the missions. I always had a suspicion that organized religion was a scam to get your money. However, I totally believed that all those pennies were going to the missions and I could not imagine the pastor keeping the money for himself. Many times in church, tears would stream down my face as it sunk in that God did indeed love me.

I did get baptized in total immersion. The floor of the altar opened up and there was a mural of a forest scene painted on the inside cover of the door that rose on hinges.

One day, while I was home meditating and feeling God's love, I marveled at how God could love me when I had messed up so many times in life. I fervently prayed and asked God, "How could you possibly love me?" God showed me a vision of the prayers I had prayed as a child where I thanked Him for each and every one of my toes. And I heard God laugh.

And He told me, "How could I not love you?"

AMENDS

My father taught me to sit on the bus facing forward. I am not one hundred percent sure that it really matters, but it is one of the very few things he taught me. So, when I can, I pick a seat that faces forward. The here and now is what I know I have. What went on in the past is only useful for instruction. Planning for the future is beneficial but none of us knows if we will be here to enjoy it, so living in the now, with our brains facing forward, seems to be a rather good idea.

I was about thirty-five when my father got in touch with me to make his amends. This was a critical time in my life since I was grappling with the pain of my second divorce. My dad had been mostly missing from my life due to his alcoholism. But at that time, he was in a program with Alcoholics Anonymous and making amends with me was his next step.

I told him frankly, "Dad, there is no way you can ever make amends for not being there when I was growing up, but there is one who made amends for you and that is Jesus Christ." I am grateful that I had it in my heart to allow my dad into my life for the last three years of his life before he died of bone cancer. I could have rejected him and accused him of not needing to come to me until he knew his death was imminent. But I chose the higher path. I decided to be better rather than bitter, and I am glad I did, because I enjoyed having that brief relationship with my dad before he died.

We were going back and forth from his apartment in Boston to my apartment in Northern New Jersey and he called very frequently. He would always start his calls saying, "Hi, this is me; is that you?" He visited me one Thanksgiving and we went to a nice restaurant. My son threw pennies into their fountain.

I was there holding my dad's hand when the death rattles occurred, and I was amazed at the fight that he had in him. I thought, "Hey, this is the stuff I am made of too."

At his funeral I wept uncontrollably as our fractured family gathered to send him off into eternity. I believe I wept more for what could have been rather than for the loss of him.

My oldest brother Jerry made all the arrangements when my dad died in 1988. Most of my siblings were there, except for my second oldest brother, Lenny, who at the time lived in Idaho and was confined to a wheelchair, and our youngest brother, Franky, who lived in a paralyzed condition in a chronic care hospital. Of the siblings, that left my younger sister Patty, my younger brother Jimmy, and my third oldest brother Freddy. I must say for a fractured family, we managed to give our dad a dignified send-off.

I recall when I was eleven and I visited my mom for my oldest brother's wedding. The reception took place back at his bride's apartment, and in the kitchen, a slight man was sobbing pitifully by the window.

"Mom," I asked, "why is that man crying?"

And she told me, "That's your father, and he's crying because you do not recognize him." I had not seen him since I was removed from my family to a foster home when I was about four. My response was to walk over to him and put my arms around him and hug him. I only knew that this was the father I longed for.

It was two years later when I saw my father again. I was visiting my mother during spring break from school and my mother brought me to see him when he was just about to leave for an Alcoholics Anonymous meeting. I remember he handed me a card with the Serenity Prayer on it and I carried it for a very long time. So, I was thirteen when I first learned the Serenity Prayer, but it was not until I was over fifty that I realized that one of the things I could never change is the past.

Around the time my father showed up in my life, I experienced a spiritual crisis. I remember listening in the balcony at church and the minister proclaimed that Christ was enough. I found myself shaking my head "no" from side to side and descending from the church balcony, believing that Christ was not enough for the pain and suffering and loss I had gone through in life. In retrospect, I was angry with God for not saving my second marriage. He could have; I knew that. But God choose not to and left me bereft. I took my anger out on God. I lost what little trust I had in Him and pretty much followed my own path which was of course folly.

I never stopped believing in God. I knew there is a God... but so does the devil. I was just so sin-sick and weak and helpless. My father being in my life at that time was an act of mercy.

It has been since 2002 that I have rededicated my life back to the Lord. All I needed was a touch from His holy hand, and I would never be the same.

Ephesians Chapter 3: verses 14-19 describes it best:

> *For this cause I bow my knees unto the Father of our lord Jesus Christ, of whom the whole family in heaven and earth is named, that He would grant you according to the riches of His glory, to be strengthened with might by His Spirit in the inner man; that Christ may dwell in your hearts by faith; and*

ye, being rooted and grounded in love may be able to comprehend with all saints what is the breadth, and length, and depth, and height; and to know the love of Christ, which passes knowledge, that you might be filled with all the fullness of God.

I understand now that it was divine wisdom that led to the dissolution of our marriage because one person cannot make a marriage. I also came to understand that what I perceived as the enemy of God attacking my marriage to destroy my soul and keep me from my heavenly home was not the main purpose of the satanic attack. At the time of the divorce, my son was four and I had dedicated him over and over in my heart to the Lord. My not being strong in the Lord and going down for the count in the fight resulted in me being negligent in consistently bringing my son up in the fear and admonishment of the Lord. To this day, my heartfelt prayer is that the Lord will lead my son back to Him.

Fathers are so important. They are the spiritual head of the family, and through their example, we get a glimpse of our heavenly Father. When that is missing, or when the father is a tyrant, it is a tough road for the child to grow and develop and have a trust in the Holy One who truly loves us.

When I fell in love with my son's father, I was so astonished! How could I love again after my heartbreaking first marriage? I could only conclude that the man had to be God. He thought he was too, but of course I figured out later that God was much more than this mere mortal. I remember, with embarrassment, the day my sister came to meet him. I went running toward her on the sidewalk and shouted, "Patty, I want you to meet God!"

I was so confused simply because I was in a reefer daze most of my free time outside of work. I suppose I was self-medicating. The other thing to understand was how much I loved my first husband Junior. I literally cried tears of blood over that man. I would cry until the tear ducts opened and mingled blood with my tears. It was a very sad marriage, mainly because he was addicted to heroin. Being able to fall in love so completely with Sammy was incredible to me.

Sammy would visit me from New York City where I lived in Cambridge and ravish me with lovemaking; yet it was more than that. He braided my hair into little braids and put me on his 6'4" inch frame and jogged with me on his shoulders from Kendall Square through Central Square and on to Harvard Square. I was crazy in love with the accent on crazy.

The purpose of me showing my scars, so to speak, is because I have very few. That is the wonder of mental illness, yet people fear it. I learned how to make it in life while my brain spills chemicals. One of the greatest strengths I have learned is keeping my mouth shut. No matter what paranoid thoughts I have, I just do not share them... especially at work.

The world has ended, and God forgot to call me to judgment. I am the only one overlooked by God. That was my delusion in my second breakdown. That is the kind of ego I have. I thought I was important enough to be the only one forgotten. That is quite a delusion. Learning to laugh at myself is a marvelous coping skill.

During my third breakdown, I was very manic and ran around the North End of Boston through Boston proper and ended up at a church volunteering to help the elderly, help children and help the needy. After I landed in Eric Lindeman Mental Health Center, I felt so much remorse at how ineffective I was to help anyone, even myself.

I like to share my experience with people who are having psychiatric problems. My true gift is that I am an encourager. In life I have met good people and bad. I think we all make choices constantly. My choice is to be like the good people. I know I have faults and weaknesses, but my strength comes from the Good Lord. It is written that "*it is not God's will that anyone perish.*"

> *The Lord is not slack concerning His promise, as some count slackness, but is longsuffering toward us, not willing that any should perish but that all should come to repentance. (2 Peter 3:9)*

If you believe that, and I do, we can only conclude that homicide and suicide are not God's will. There have been times in life when I was suicidal and times when my emotions ran strong enough for me to seek help for homicidal feelings. It is terrible when your own emotions frighten you. For me, the homicidal feelings signaled my healing, because suicidal tendencies tempted me up until my late twenties. During my pregnancy, when I was twenty-nine, I had a lot of disturbing aggressive feelings. It was very distressing. Of course, I had stopped taking all medications while I was pregnant, and smoking was repugnant to me. Somehow, I waddled through the nine months and delivered a wonderful son.

I managed to stay off medication until my son was three and a half and I had a psychotic episode that landed me in Bellevue. At the time, my marriage was so bad that my husband did not even realize I was taking care of his son while I was in the middle of psychosis. I was so far gone that the doctors at the hospital were talking about confining me to a mental hospital for the rest of my life. Mysteriously, I suddenly understood what they were talking about and explicitly outlined to them the torturous things my husband had been putting me through. The doctors turned their gaze from me to him, wondering who the one who ought to be confined was. In a week I was home, but my husband told me he wanted a divorce. The news hit me hard. From his point of view, I guess it was difficult being married to a psychotic. I know I would not want my son to be in love with someone who was mentally unstable. These are the kinds of things one must admit when they are a few French fries short of a Happy Meal.

So, I found myself a single parent with a mental handicap who had to find her way in the world. My reaction was anger toward God. I knew He could have intervened and changed the situation, but He did not choose to do that. So, I was on my own. I believed in Him but I did not think He was enough.

I reverted to dabbling in the occult. I even had the audacity to pray the "Our Father" before I read the tarot. Interestingly, my readings were accurate, but I realize now that was the deception that kept me bound to delve deeper into the occult. I became very expert at casting horoscopes until it was announced that sidereal calculations were replacing tropical calculations. Then, I sort of caught on. The whole thing was poppycock and an enormous waste of time. I realized the presumptuousness of even thinking that I could figure out what the position of the planets meant.

A friend of mine visited me from the West Coast in the early 90s. He shared with me that he did not really want to accept my hospitality even though he was hard-pressed to pay for his own hotel accommodations. He told me that he was surprised with all my dabbling in the occult that God had not given me up to be a reprobate. He showed me the famous passages in the book of Romans

(Romans 1:28) that predicted reprobation would be the result when people followed their own crooked way even after they knew the truth.

Somehow, I was protected. I look back now and realize God was watching over me even while I was in rebellion. After my friend talked to me about the danger of my dabbling in the occult, I ended up gathering up my crystal ball and my tarot deck wrapped in silk in its nice wooden hand-carved box together with all my astrological books and tossed them in a faraway garbage can.

I remember distinctly the sensation of my head being gonged with the goings-on of the planets moving in my mind. I was at work and I was having a difficult time focusing on my word processing job because of the manifestation of reverberations in my head. I knew I was doing the right thing renouncing the occult, but I was still a long way from the point where I rededicated my life to Christ. That happened fourteen years later. In the meantime, I still indulged in my wicked pot habit and inconvenient lovers. These were men I unconsciously gravitated toward to work out my abandonment issues.

It is clear to me now that all my life I was looking for my daddy's love. After all, I was bereft of him since I was four years old. I remember him carrying me on his shoulders when he took me home from the hospital after I cut my toes in the fountain at Blackstone Park in South Boston. How ironic that my son's father carried me on his shoulders through Cambridge when I was twenty-six years old. My daddy fracture is very painful, yet I know that I have a heavenly Father who is perfect and able, and I am willing to trust Him. Trusting God is the best decision I ever made in my life even though I waited until I was fifty-three to make that decision.

My path has been fraught with many trials and tribulations. I have survived them all, but not without emotional scars, bruises, and damage. I have been crushed but not destroyed.

My erroneous thinking that Jesus was not enough was just that: a terrible error. My faith during the time of my divorce was not strong enough but I thank God that my faith is becoming stronger. Since the Lord revealed himself to me and gave me a touch of His holy hand where I experienced His unfathomable love, I have consciously decided to trust the Lord no matter what. After close to two decades of renewed determination to follow the Lord, I can heartily conclude, "God is more than enough." When they sing in church that "God's Grace is Enough," my shout is… "more than enough!"

EXERCISING DEMOCRACY

I angrily banged the nails in the chair, trying to repair it, and all the time I was thinking of my nemesis that my ex-husband had betrayed me with. I could not pound the nails in hard enough. There was no outlet for my anger and my rage was consuming.

Around that time, I received a notice that my rent was scheduled to be doubled and a hearing date had been set to dispute it. The shock of this threw me into a frenzy. I was on the bus obsessing and fuming over the fact of how unfair it was that I lived in a rent-controlled apartment and the officials of the town had, by stapling a document to the rent control order, allowed the landlord to double the rent for "Substantial Rehabilitation Improvements." Then I had a thought, "Hey, I am not in this alone; not only does this ordinance affect me but also the other twenty-five tenants in my building as well as everyone else in a rent-controlled apartment in the town of West New York, New Jersey."

I went to work the next day and during my break period made up a poster on a plain sheet of paper. It announced the ordinance and the hearing date. I ran off the flyer on the company's copier. At that time, I worked for advertising marketeers who ran the business from the company's dining room in the owner's brownstone building on the Upper East Side of Manhattan. The copier along with filing cabinets, shelves, and postage meter were housed in the basement. There were three advertising sales representatives who worked with the principal owner upstairs under the dining room chandelier. I was the office manager and at that time there were no other clerical workers.

I stood in Port Authority, where a stream of people boarded the bus back to West New York, and handed out my poster which warned the people of the doubling of the rents and how we needed to organize, protect ourselves, and protest at the hearing. I then contacted the New Jersey Tenants Organization (NJTO) who sent representatives to talk to our tenants and brought pamphlets letting us know what our rights were.

The town I lived in was on the west side of the Hudson River overlooking the New York skyline from the New Jersey side. It was a bedroom community of New York City. With the increased demand for housing, it was dubbed "the Gold Coast." I had a two-bedroom apartment and walked up four flights to the five-story building. From my living room, I had a treasured view of the New York skyline.

The tenants of the town had a court date to address the ordinance. It was an exciting night for me. I was not alone. The courtroom was full. A staff of court officers surrounded the judge at the front of the courtroom. Arturo led his building's tenants, and I led mine. Bobby led his building and there were several other buildings represented by their tenants. Somehow, I caught the eye of Joyce, who was in court from the nearby town of Weehawken, and we became friends at first sight. We waved to each other across the courtroom from our courthouse pews.

I was very impressed when Bobby got up to represent his building. He was articulate and straight to the point as to why the doubling of the rents was unfair to the tenants. Immediately I wanted to befriend him. I was refreshingly surprised by his intelligent personality. Arturo also had the bravado of all his tenants edging him on and applauding him. I got up and asked, "What good is it if we have new windows, doors, and cabinets if we cannot afford to put food in those cabinets?" I heard one of the court officers gasp.

Later, I found Joyce sitting on the hallway bench of the courthouse. She had a bad headache and I offered her aspirin. Joyce declined. She was too wise to take aspirin from someone she did not know well.

A few days later, Joyce planned to visit me in my fourth-floor walk-up apartment bringing with her a few tenant activists from Weehawken. We sat in my living room and she told me, "You are the only one who can organize the tenants of West New York." I responded with incredulity.

"Are you kidding me? I struggle to find my socks in the morning to get to work on time."

"No," she insisted, "I saw you in Port Authority handing out the flyers to get the people to go to court to fight the issue of substantial rehabilitation. Only a leader would do that and only you can organize the tenants of West New York." When they told me the story of how rent-controlled tenants had their buildings set on fire to make way for gentrification in the neighboring town of Hoboken, I relented. NJTO put me in touch with Jennifer Brooks to represent us for a minimal fee. The tenants of the various buildings in town chipped in and we retained her to represent us.

On that first night in the court I had failed to note the building address Bobby represented. I knew it was important to find him. In order to find Bobby, I went from building to building in our town looking for him and finally found him. He was a tireless worker for our cause.

So, with Joyce's help, the help of our attorney Jennifer Brooks, and the others, the United Tenants of West New York Association was formed. We used the slogan, "IN UNITY THERE IS STRENGTH." We appointed a tenant of another building, a well-known union leader, as our president. We elected Arturo as treasurer, my next-door neighbor, Lorenzo, as sergeant of arms, and I was elected secretary. We successfully united most of the rent-controlled buildings in our town.

On one occasion, my five-year-old son played with his cars on the floor of the mayor's office while the mayor gave audience to me as I expressed our concerns and need for places to meet. The mayor sat behind a huge desk and we talked while he handled multiple tasks over the telephone. He told me he was behind what the tenants were doing but warned me that I had to play by his rules or else he would spread the rumor that I was a communist. His wife came into the room and burst into tears when I retorted, "If you do that, I'll have my five brothers put on their military uniforms and march down Boulevard East." I heard my own false bravado and I tried my best to diffuse the situation. I fluffed up his ego because I needed the mayor to give us venues for our meetings.

The mayor helped us in our efforts. He gave us permission to use Hudson Hall and to have a rally in the park. At the park gathering, I had my friend from church sing the national anthem. She had a wonderfully gifted voice. We gathered all the townspeople together and we each gave our speeches. Joyce got up and said, "I am tired of being pushed around, I am tired of the injustice, I am tired of having to fight for our rights!" Then Sid, an older man who was from the neighboring town of North Bergen, boomed out in his well-spoken voice how it was our right to have affordable housing and our right to have quiet enjoyment of the property we rented. Joyce pointed out that although we lived in rented apartments, they actually were our homes. We were all in agreement and kept the community notified of every court date. Because I had advertising experience, I knew to get the local press involved and they did give us coverage.

We had a meeting at the Knights of Columbus Hall. Arturo and I were the speakers. I got up before the gathering to share the plight of one of the tenants who lived in my building. He had died of an aneurism when he found out his rent was doubling. He worked in a deli and was the father of two small boys. His wife took in penny piece work of embroidery to help with the food bill. While I was giving my speech, I suddenly got panicky and started tilting over to one side. I could hardly keep myself upright, and Arturo, sensing my discomfit and calamity, reached over to help steady me to stand straight. I had sensed the animosity of some of the people in the gathering. It was obvious to me that not all attendees were supportive of us.

On one court night, we had people marching around the courthouse chanting in Spanish, "No aumente la renta" (don't raise the rent). I remember that cool autumn night in particular because the judge acted totally baffled that we had managed to make such a noise in the bedroom community of West New York, New Jersey. My friend Bobby burst into the courtroom and loudly railed at the landlord's attorney, saying, "Jakowski, how many people have you made homeless! You are heartless!"

Jakowski was not his real name, of course, but he became the focus of my rage. One night, while reflecting on my memory of the Bible verse that said "Pray for your enemies" [Matthew 5:43-45], I forced against all my will to pray for him. Interestingly, during one court session where I took the stand, Jakowski announced to the judge that he wanted it to go on record that whether or not the tenants could afford the increase in rent was immaterial and should not be mentioned. The judge agreed that no one called to the witness stand could mention that affordability was an issue. So Jakowski asked a few questions and then provoked me with the comment on the photographs I had presented to the court showing the defects in the workmanship. He asked sneeringly, "How come you didn't take any pictures of all the things that were right and show only the things that are wrong?"

I answered swiftly and surely, much to his consternation, "Because I couldn't afford the film." He looked pitifully at the judge, but the judge allowed the statement on the record.

This rent control battle went on for two and a half years and ended in 1985. There were many meetings in different tenants' apartments, including my own. I remember bringing my six-year-old son with me to one meeting where I handed him a Rubik's Cube to play with. He came to me with it solved and I beamed in admiration, but then I realized that he had simply peeled off the paper squares and placed them in the right places. He had solved the puzzle that way!

In the end, we did manage to outlaw substantial rehabilitation in the town of West New York, but the tenants of my building were exempt from the protection since the landlord had already made the improvements. Because of this *ipso facto* regulation, the tenants of our building had to pay the double amount of rent. And, if people vacated the apartments, the landlord would be allowed to triple the rent. During our battle we had placed our rents in an escrow account. Our attorney told us that an anonymous benefactor had paid the difference between the doubled rent and the previous rent for all the tenants in our building for the two-and-a-half-year period we had fought in court. We grumbled about our defeat while feeling truly fortunate over the generosity of the mysterious benefactor.

Over the years, most of the rent-controlled buildings in the town were converted to condominiums or cooperatives, but the elderly and disabled tenants in those and other rent-controlled buildings were allowed to stay at the rent-controlled rates. A few buildings remain rent-controlled to this day.

A few years later, I realized that during my third nervous breakdown, which had occurred a decade earlier, I showed up at a church where they were asking for community volunteers. I was twenty-four at the time and I lived in Boston. I was in the middle of decomposing, running around the North End of Boston, and I had just finished handing out teabags to attendees of a funeral milling about the outside of a funeral parlor. I was very manic and had signed up at the church to volunteer for all types of roles. While I was recovering in the hospital, I felt so much remorse because I really wanted to keep those promises but was in no condition to do so.

Ten years later, I was thirty-five when I became a tenant activist. Without realizing it, by fighting for tenant's rights for two and a half years, I had unwittingly fulfilled the promises I made while in a manic state many years before. I feel humbly grateful that I had that opportunity to keep those promises.

BOBBY

"I'm home," Bobby would announce every time he arrived at my apartment. We had become good friends. He taught me how he steamed broccoli and we would have Sunday dinner together. We were close like brother and sister. He trusted me with his house keys to water his plants when he traveled to South America. He was super intelligent and fluent in at least two languages. He was younger than me. We had a lot of counterpoint thoughts. He had no use for my Jesus and was an advocate of Seth from the book *Seth Speaks* by Jane Roberts. I was in the New Age mystical period of my life where I would read the tarot, cast horoscopes, and read palms. Weirdly, my readings were mostly accurate.

We would walk together on Saturday mornings and go to breakfast. My good friend Maria would watch my seven-year-old son when we did this. One day as we were walking, Bobby suddenly turned to me in consternation and blurted out that he had had a dream about me. He told me that in the dream, he had died and his friends at the gravesite read a letter from me in which I declared that he had taken the Eucharist while he was in the hospital dying. He raised his voice and said, "That doesn't represent me at all; belief in Jesus does not represent me. There I was dying, and they gave me the Eucharist and I did not know what I was doing."

Whereupon, I replied, "Bobby, I didn't do that. That was a dream." So, he calmed down and we talked about things like helping elderly people cross the street and doing good deeds.

He linked arms with me, grinned, and said, "Here we are, two prominent citizens of West New York, walking down Bergenline Avenue." Then we went on to enjoy breakfast in a nice Cuban restaurant.

Bobby and I each had a writer's germ and we would talk about our different ideas for writing. He worked for the telephone company which was splitting up into subsidiaries. The title for his book would be, *Ma Bell and the Seven Little Chimes*.

He took me to the office building where he worked one Fourth of July and we watched the fireworks in the luxury of a good view. When we left the building, we were each handed a bunch of balloons in the lobby. We passed out the balloons as we walked through Times Square back to Port Authority to catch our bus to New

Jersey. We laughed and chatted with the passers-by who took our balloons.

He came to visit me at my job where I worked as the administrative assistant for the director of construction in a new high-rise building they had erected. Bobby walked into the lobby, looked around at all the green marble, and remarked in mock astonishment, "Oh, Oz!"

After our tenant battle, Bobby's building went condo. He sold his apartment and moved back to New York, buying a new apartment in Brooklyn. I visited him there with my boyfriend and he seemed very happy. We kept in touch with each other but there was a period of time when we got out of touch.

A couple of years after my building doubled its rent, I found a house I could buy. I moved into that house with a broken foot which is another story and realized that I had not heard from Bobby and that he wasn't answering any of my calls. So, I wrote him a long letter because he was a friend that I greatly valued and did not want to lose touch with him.

I got a call one day at work from Bobby's mother telling me that he was in the hospital dying of AIDS. She told me that she had read my letter telling Bobby all the escapades I had gone through since I had last heard from him. She told me that he was having her read the same letter over and over again because he had liked it so much. Then she asked me, "Would you please send another letter to him so she would have something different to read?"

During our conversation, she also mentioned to me that he had taken Holy Communion.

I thought hard about what to write. I wrote about what a good person I thought he was and how he continued to fight alongside the tenants long after his building had turned into a condominium and how unselfish and loyal he was in his fight for tenants' rights. I wrote how sorry I was that he was sick and that I was praying for him. I wrote how I knew that he was always sincere in all he did and since I knew that about him, I knew he had taken Holy Communion in sincerity. With a few other things mentioned, I mailed the letter to his mother. I stopped into Times Square Church and filled out prayer cards for his recovery.

Not long after, I heard of his death. He was only thirty-three. I was devastated by his death because I did love Bobby as a brother. I had wanted him to be my friend for the rest of my life, but now this heartfelt desire was thwarted. I was livid with rage for several months. I was not angry at anyone in particular, just angry that I no longer had my friend.

I went to his dignified memorial service, using a cane to assist my foot that had been broken. About a week later I heard from Bobby's mother again. She told me that at the gravesite with Bobby's friends, they read my letter and put it in his pocket to be buried with him.

After I got off the phone, I suddenly remembered the day he had scolded me over the dream he had of me linking him to Jesus because he took Holy Communion. To this day, I do not know how he knew I would write that letter through a dream that happened three years before he died.

The only way I can reconcile this mystery in my mind is to think that the enemy of God wanted to thwart Bobby from turning to Jesus. But then, I imagine Bobby showing up in the afterlife with all the glowing recommendations in the letter about him being the caring, loving person Bobby had portrayed in life.

My hope to this day is that when my assignment here on Earth is finished, I will find my friend Bobby in heaven.

THE AMERICAN SCREAM

My son was about nine and I had him join Cub Scouts. The meeting was held in a reformed church. I became his den mother and worked along with Ruth and Marco for a couple of years. Marco was a lot of fun and we enjoyed working with the boys together. I would tell him how I prayed on my way to work in New York City from New Jersey every day and he would laugh about how I was going into the "sin" city and the irony of me praying while on my way there. Although I was backslidden, I still prayed.

Ruth and I were on friendly terms too. Ruth was having a difficult time selling her house. She convinced me to come over to look at it. I fell in love with the house immediately. It was a little house with a porch and three bedrooms. It was at a very low price, but I still couldn't afford it and only had a couple of thousand dollars in an

IRA. So, the broker, the lawyer, and the bank worked with me to give me a "quick and easy" loan.

I shared with my son that I remembered we had prayed for a house with a tree in the back yard and this house had a tree in front. And he told me, "Ma, you prayed for a tree, but I prayed for a swimming pool." The house came with an above ground pool in the back yard.

After my dad died, my oldest brother, Jerry, handed me a couple of thousand dollars to help me with the closing. A couple of friends loaned me some money because I could not qualify for the mortgage if I had outstanding debt. On the day of the closing, I was on my way to the bank to get a certified check. As I was coming down the stairs, I fell on a broken step.

After my trip to the hospital in an ambulance, I lay on a gurney in the hallway of the emergency room for several hours. I went into delirium and started laughing maniacally. Along came a doctor and looked at my foot which was almost on backward. She took two pillows, put my foot in the middle, and twisted my foot back in place. I was in a hospital in North Bergen, but I screamed so loud, I think I could have been heard at the George Washington Bridge which was a few towns down the Hudson River. Perhaps the doctor saved my foot, but she did not use any pain medication and that was brutal.

Now I ended up signing for my house while I was still on the gurney on my way to the operating room to get my foot screwed back together. I hesitated only for a moment but decided as an act of faith I had to believe I would be able to walk again, and that I must sign for the house. So, while I was on my sickbed in the hospital, I signed all the papers for my mortgage on my new home.

My friend Arturo came and took pictures of my foot in the cast. The landlord stopped in to visit me. I called a well-known personal injury attorney; he also visited me in the hospital and told me I did all the right things for the case.

Ruth and her family took care of my son for a few days while I was in the hospital. When they headed for their new home in Florida, they left my son with a neighbor in my old building for the remainder of my hospital stay. While I was in the hospital, I called to see how much of a disability payment I could receive. I found out that because I worked in New York City and lived in New Jersey that I only qualified for $150 per month. I was stymied. I had a mortgage of $1,300 per month and I had used just about all my savings for the down payment and closing on the house. Obviously, I could not return to work right away, so where would I get my next mortgage payment?

My neighbor came to get me, stopped off to pick up a wheelchair, and brought me to my new home. I climbed the stairs up the porch on my rear end. My son came home, and his two friends came by to play. All my furniture was back in the old apartment. The sellers of my property had left a bed and a couch. I had no refrigerator and would send my son out to buy ice to keep the milk cold. My son and his two friends swam merrily in the above ground swimming pool in the back yard. I tried to stay calm in the grip of my financial dilemma. I decided I would refuse to worry and trust God. It was the only thing I could do to stay sane.

In my backslidden state, I was not going to church and I was not reading the Bible. I knew instinctively that if I did not depend on God in my current circumstances that I would literally go stark raving mad. I could not go mad because I had an eleven-year-old boy to take care of. So, I prayed and buried myself in novels and knitting and refused to worry. This went on for three weeks until I learned from my job during a telephone call that they had decided to pay me a full salary while I took as long as I needed to recover. "The Lord is my shepherd; I shall not want..." [Psalm 23]. That is provision.

A week later, Maria's daughter took a day off from work to pack up my stuff in the old apartment and send a moving van with all my furniture to my new home.

I paid all my bills, but my credit cards were doing a shuffle. Two years later, I got a nice check for the accident caused by my previous landlord's neglect to fix the broken stair I had fallen on. I immediately paid off twenty thousand dollars in credit card debt. After that, it occurred to me that I was over my head at the rate of ten thousand dollars per year — just the amount of interest I paid on the mortgage.

We lived in the house with my dog, Jesse, who was part Doberman Pincer and German Shepherd (and I think part teddy bear) along with our four cats: Powder, Puff, Princess Fluffy, and Horowitz. I had Jesse and the two Creamsicle-colored cats Powder and Puff before I moved to the house. My son had found a little sick cat in the street we named Crystal, but when we brought her to the vet, she had to be put to sleep. While we were at the vet, we acquired Princess Fluffy who was a gorgeous angora calico cat. Princess Fluffy had a litter of kittens and we kept her son, Horowitz.

Fortunately, the house had a pet door, so we were all content until not-so-friendly neighborhood kids started coming through the pet door to steal from us. I suppose they must have given our dog a hamburger because we were robbed seven times in eight years!

I came home one day, and a group of boys were washing my white shingled house down for me. They were my son's new friends. He liked the game Dungeons and Dragons and had posted a sign in a local comic bookstore to meet friends of the same interests. The boys all hung around our house for the time we lived there. They came to me one day and asked me if they could build a skateboard ramp. And me, not having a clue to what they were really asking said, "Yes." So, they started coming into the house with sheets of plywood and huge electric saws they had borrowed from their parents, and the next thing I knew, my entire back yard was filled with a giant skateboard contraption. (I had previously removed the swimming pool after a couple of years in the house because I had feared accidents happening while I was at work.)

There I would be, reading a book while listening to the thump, thump of the neighborhood boys on the skateboard ramp as they learned to become expert skateboarders. I would sigh and think, "Someday this will all be gone," and that thought would give me the patience to tolerate the noise. There were many empty pizza boxes in those days.

Financially I was about ten thousand dollars a year over my head. I lived modestly, I never owned a car, and I was thrifty enough to squeeze a penny until it cried. But the figures just didn't work. I realized after year six that I had to sell the house, so I put the property up for sale. In two years' time, not one person ever came to look at the property. This was in 1994 and in my area the housing market was a bust.

At the time, I worked for a stock market trader and a lawyer out of the trader's brownstone building in New York City. I brought my problem to work and both men I worked for tried to negotiate with the bank for a doable mortgage. I had an adjustable rate mortgage and the interest zoomed up to over nine percent. I tried to refinance with a fixed rate, but my debt ratio did not allow a refinance.

Many of the original fixings in the house were cosmetic. The house needed repairs that were estimated to be at least twenty thousand dollars which I did not have. I was under water and in over my head. After reeling from the instability, which was like walking on a funhouse floor, I realized that I was not born with a house on my back. Since I decided there was no way a house was going to put me in the grave, I found a lawyer to help me go bankrupt and foreclose.

I had put a lot of my earnings into that house and came up with zilch. The sellers were compensated, the real estate broker and selling attorney were compensated, but I had zilch.

My major problem was my pets. After my foreclosure, who would rent to someone with a teenage son, a dog, and four cats? I prayed fervently for a home for my pets. I knew I could not pick one over the other to take to a rental apartment. One day, out of the blue, I got the idea to call my town hall to ask for help. I talked to a fellow who steered me to Candy who owned her own pet grooming store. He thought Candy would be able to help me. I told my story to Candy on the phone and she said to me, "You can't separate those animals; they are bonded." I thought of my own family and how we were all separated, and I started to cry, and I told her how the government took me away from my family when I was only four. Candy was so moved that she decided to take all four cats herself. And she found a home for my teddy bear dog, Jesse.

The lady came over and gave her a biscuit and Jesse went with her. Jesse knew she had to have a home because she had heard me say to my son, "If I don't find a home for Jesse, I will have to bring her to an animal shelter."

And then Jesse had turned around, and I swear I heard her say, "What?" Well, you would have had to be there.

I think it is extraordinary that my prayers for homes for my pets were answered. My dog was eight years old and the cats, except for Horowitz, were close to Jesse's age.

I found an apartment for me and my son and turned the house back to the bank. I have not had any pets since. Even though that was over twenty years ago, I still miss them.

It was in 1996 that I went through bankruptcy and foreclosure. When the financial crisis hit America in 2008, I was very aware of the quick and easy loans that had been handed out to anyone who could fog up a mirror. In horror I listened to the news as it was reported that banks were being given **billions** of dollars to tide them over their bad investments. I could not believe this was happening and that we were giving our tax money to banks because they had made bad investments. I could understand why Fannie Mae and Freddie Mac might need to be bailed out because they had backed up all those mortgages. But didn't that mean that the banks were the ones who were protected by those mortgages that were insured by them? Then there was the talk about the investments the banks made in derivatives. I came to believe that those derivatives were investments of bundled up quick and easy mortgages. Really? Who was going to bail out the individual taxpayers for any bad investments they had made?

Dare I mention homeless mothers and children and homeless veterans?

So, it turns out the American scream is really more of a whimper.

THE IMPACT OF 9/11

Everyone was impacted by the terror attack of 9/11; for me, it was a pivotal point in my life. My day started out as a typical workday. I arrived at Port Authority on a beautiful September morning and decided to walk up Eighth Avenue from 42nd Street to my job on 53rd Street. As usual, I was half-asleep since my coffee had not fully kicked in. I had walked four blocks when I stepped off the curb and quickly jumped back to avoid getting hit by a fire truck on its way to the disaster. Two other trucks whizzed by as my heart raced from almost being hit by the first truck. Not knowing what had happened, I continued to my workplace and found a large number of people gathered in the lobby craning up their necks to watch a television hung on the wall. The first plane had hit and as I stood there, the second plane crashed into the World Trade Center Tower. I numbly took the elevator up to the seventh floor where I worked as an administrative assistant.

The whole group of people in my department was in a turmoil trying to piece together what was happening. Then we heard on the radio that a plane had hit the Pentagon. We started talking about how we would sleep on the floor of our office for the night when I got a call from my friend Joyce who also worked in New York City. Joyce wanted to meet me to accompany her home. All the tunnels and bridges were closed, and she had to get back to New Jersey because she was diabetic and needed her insulin and she heard that a ferry could take us across the river. I agreed to meet her at Burger King, across from Port Authority at 42nd Street. She would walk there from 23rd Street and I would walk from 53rd Street and Seventh Avenue.

I walked back the few blocks to Burger King feeling very surreal; I was not understanding what was happening and feeling like the world was coming to an end. I had to wait for Joyce and started praying while I was waiting. For the first time I ever could remember, Burger King was closed in the middle of the morning. I sat outside on the pavement and I kept praying fervently. I remember feeling something like a piece of rice being planted into my heart, a seed of hope, or perhaps blessed assurance. Joyce showed up and neither of us knew what was happening but we stopped for a slice of pizza and headed toward the docks to catch the ferry back to New Jersey.

The line at the ferry was exceedingly long. There were people there who had escaped from the debris and rubble which was still on them. We were in line with people suffering from the shock of seeing people falling out of the towers and their own close call with death. Patiently, we moved slowly toward the ferry. It took several hours for our turn to board. We arrived safely on the Jersey side and walked the dozen blocks to Joyce's house. There were no cars on Boulevard East. A few police cars were parked intermittently in the middle of the Boulevard to ward off traffic. We saw the smoke rising across the river from the devastated towers.

At the time this disaster occurred I was still backslidden. It would be several months before my encounter with the Savior who touched me with His holy hand, delivering love. So, even though I had given up astrology a dozen years before, my curious instinct was to look to the stars to figure things out. It was a few days after 9/11 that I picked up a current astrology magazine and while I was reading an article, I became thoroughly disgusted. The writer was stating that God was both good and evil. I knew that was a lie because I know that God is good. I flung the book and threw it away, realizing the underlying twisted danger of astrology in mixing truth and lies.

For about three weeks, people gathered in churches. Although I lived next door to a church, I did not go. I stayed in and watched television programs. I watched one where President Bush recited the Lord's Prayer with the members of Congress and other dignitaries. I caught my breath when he finished the Lord's Prayer, thinking for a split second that we could actually enter a period of world peace and then I heard him say: "Let's go to war."

I continued to move about as usual, walking around as if in the middle of a nightmare. I noticed that the firehouse where the trucks had whizzed by me on that fateful day had signs up showing that none of those men had returned. The whole country was in mourning and I mourned with them. I mourned particularly for those children who had lost their parents. Still, a bus driver complimented me for being able to smile my customary greeting to him. A few weeks later, from my home, I could see the two columns of lights that were streaming up in the night sky, filling in the void of the towers.

The impact of 9/11 interfered with the real estate concerns of my company and I lost my job. I was eligible for unemployment insurance and decided that I could use the time to recover from my emotional weariness. I took a course updating my computer skills; this kept me busy.

My encounter with the Lord occurred about nine months after 9/11. I did quit smoking pot after that, as He had commanded, but I floundered about how I was to proceed in my new walk with Christ. Although I lived next door to a church, I did not think that church was the one I should necessarily go to. So, I looked for a sign from the Lord to direct me.

One day while leaving computer school, it was pouring rain. The receptionist, Isabel, offered me a ride home which I gratefully accepted. We were talking in the car and she was telling me she went to the church next door to where I lived. I told her I had visited her church but was put off by the people who fell on the floor. "Oh, that is the Holy Spirit," she told me. "The Holy Spirit acts differently on each person. For instance, I find that the Holy Spirit brings me to tears." When she said that to me, I suddenly recalled the early days when I first went to church after being saved. I would frequently have tears streaming down my face as I learned that God loved me. When she said that to me, I realized I had not understood that the Holy Spirit was working on me. The impact of her conversation made me agree to go to her church.

The day I walked in, I felt the gentle guiding of the Holy Spirit to the pew where Isabel sat with her two little boys. From the back of the church, I was unable to detect that it was her and when I was guided to her seat, that was all the sign I needed to know this was where the Lord wanted me. That day an altar call was made, and I rededicated my life to the Lord. The sister in Christ who talked to me after I did that realized I had testimony and needed counseling. She introduced me to Eve who is the founder of Solid Foundation Ministry. I entered counseling to be healed by the power of the Lord of all my past confusions and sins. The most important thing I learned was forgiveness — not only of those who had victimized me, but forgiveness of myself for my own faults and sins.

One lady I talked with at the church told me that she had worked in the Twin Towers but on the day of the disaster, she had stayed home sick. There were many testimonies at that time of similar stories.

I continued in the church and the Lord cleaned me up quite a bit. One day, a minister with a healing anointing visited our church. A call was made for anyone who had a need for healing to go to the altar to receive prayer. Although I had a few minor aches and pains, I declined the offer, realizing how busy the minister was, and decided to stay in my pew and pray for the man of God. As I prayed, I suddenly felt grit in my mouth coming from my teeth. I moved the grit from my tongue to my fingers and realized that the Holy Spirit was removing the built-up plaque from my teeth. It astonished me that the Lord would clean my teeth. Since I was still out of work, I had neglected to go to the dentist, but the Lord saw my need of dental work and took care of it

One Sunday evening, the pastor's son gave a discourse that unpacked the following Bible verse [Mark 4:1]:

> *Again, Jesus began to teach by the lake. The crowd that gathered around him was so large that he got into a boat and sat in it out on the lake, while all the people were along the shore at the water's edge.*

He pointed out that while the crowd was content to stand at the shore of the water's edge, there are some that want to be closer to the Lord and swim out to the boat to be nearer to Jesus. I want to be right there in the boat with Him!

OVERCOMING SMOKE

Pastor railed against false idols and challenged those of us in the congregation to give up our idols. He vehemently threw a pack of cigarettes in a garbage can that was in front of the altar. Next, he flung and broke a statue of the Virgin Mary which upset me. After all, I had been brought up Catholic and still harbor a deep love for Mother Mary. He told us he wanted us to go home and think about our idols and then return to church in the evening and bring our idols along with us and put them in the garbage can.

I spent the afternoon mentally wrestling with myself. I was conflicted by his breaking the statue of the Blessed Virgin. It was as if someone had spit on the flag of the United States of America! But, I knew deep down that I really was addicted to nicotine. The battle was whether I would never return to church or if I would bring my two unfinished packs of cigarettes to church and put my idol of cigarettes into the garbage pail at the front of the altar.

It had been about six months since I had quit smoking pot. Quitting pot was just a decision I made after Jesus told me that "the pot has got to go." It did not involve the withdrawal that I knew from experience ceasing nicotine would cause. Six months before, I had rededicated my life to Christ and my soul's success depended upon the outcome of that afternoon's wrestle.

I prayed feverishly, and I felt the Holy Spirit comforting me softly, saying that to honor Mary is to honor the Lord. I knew that Mary is not a statue. That part of the argument being settled, and my feeling vindicated for my love of Mary, I was able to decide to quit smoking cigarettes.

So that night, I put my two unfinished packs of cigarettes in the pail at the front of the altar and put down my idol of smoking altogether.

I had access to the internet, so I joined a smoking cessation blog where we encouraged each other daily with platitudes such as, "I love to breathe."

During my withdrawal, I had to use every tool available. I prayed, "Dear Lord, help me crave you more than I crave nicotine." I have been nicotine-free since December 2002, but it was not easy.

One of the tools I used was to round up all my splintered-off personalities. I do not have multiple personalities per se but there are parts of me that have been arrested at certain ages of trauma. I found it beneficial to round up all these splintered-off selves and put them in an imaginary circle and try to get all these different parts of myself to cooperate! This went on for weeks. The best thing I had going for me at the time was that I was unemployed and did not need to bring my nicotine fits into the workplace.

I tried reasoning with myself. After all, I thought, I have a compulsive eating habit and a smoking habit but if I give up smoking, I will only have to work on the overeating issue. Little did I know then that there is so much more work needed with the eating habit that likes to push down from my consciousness my tendencies to manipulate and my integrity faults along with all the other painful facts and feelings I like to deny and run away from such as my stubbornness and my innate desire to have my own way.

I psychoanalyzed myself and concluded that my fascination with cigarettes went all the way back to when my brothers stole cartons of them to buy us food. I recalled how I loved candy cigarettes and even the ones that you did not eat but that puffed powder. Well, that was during the 50s and then there were so many commercials on television as to how popular and unique you were if you smoked.

For the life of me I cannot recall when I smoked my first real cigarette. Since my memory is insufficient, I can only conclude that it must be a repressed memory. I do not recall smoking before I was twelve years old. Then,

I would go to the store and buy my foster mother her cigarettes. I would put them on her tab at the little grocery store. No one noticed when I put her brand on the tab for myself. I smoked with the seventh-graders, who I fit in with, but I cannot say that any meaningful friendships developed beyond our mutual getting away with acting like we were big.

While I was incarcerated for a year, cigarettes were used to control the inmates. This went for Charles Street Jail, the Youth Service Board, the House of Good Shepherd, and the Lancaster Reform School. I regard this kind of control as criminal, but I suppose it was the most convenient way to control the rebellious inmates of these institutions.

When I ran away from reform school, I quickly relished my cigarette habit to the degree that I was smoking three packs of cigarettes a day at age fifteen. Cigarettes in the late 60s cost only thirty-five cents a pack. During this point in time, at a party I was offered pot. I tried it, felt the music dancing on top of my head, and liked it very much. So, my pot habit and my smoking habit were somewhat entwined. I am grateful that pot was the worse drug in my circle of acquaintances at the time because I do not think I would have had the good sense to turn a harder drug down. At one time, I did get access to bennies, but after washing the ceiling in the middle of the night, I knew I had to get away from them.

When I was twenty-nine and became pregnant, I could not smoke. My body would not tolerate cigarettes. I stayed smoke-free for nineteen months until a friend who was a coffee and cigarette buddy came to visit me in New Jersey from her home in Boston. All it took was one cigarette to get me smoking again for the next twenty-two years. There were times I tried to quit but I would find myself leaving the house to buy cigarettes at two in the morning at a nearby bar. It was a disgusting habit, but I didn't want to leave it any more than I wanted to leave my pot habit.

So, I was fifty-three when I finally overcame my smoking habit. I had tapered down to smoking only three packs a week when I decided to quit but it was still an ordeal that left me cranky. I know some people get delivered from nicotine immediately. But, when I think of it, I had my chance of deliverance from nicotine when I easily quit during pregnancy. That was not the case in my future struggles to quit smoking. I learned the hard way that one cigarette is a pack of lies. That is why I am adamant that I will never allow myself to smoke again: not pot or cigarettes! After all, my body is the temple of the Holy Spirit.

PRETEND YOU ARE NORMAL

The strange thing about pretending you are normal is that if you do it long enough, you actually become normal. Then you realize we live in a crazy world to begin with and being normal puts you in the minority. That being stated, if you are willing to learn from a woman with a history of mental illness, then this is a course in the right direction.

My first diagnosis was acute schizophrenia (I was nineteen at the time). A year later, I was told that I was manic-depressive. Two years later, I was diagnosed as bipolar. My next diagnosis after a severe break and subsequent suicide attempt was opposite pole disease and associated schizophrenia (when do I get my degree?). The last diagnosis I had was major affective disorder.

One of the first things about pretending you are normal is to try to "look" sane. Exactly what that means of course is optional depending on the circumstances. For instance, if you want a job, it is better to show up for the interview looking your Sunday best. This might mean wearing stockings if you are a lady (no, not just stockings) or letting your Mohawk grow out if you are a guy. The rules change constantly, but neat and clean always looks pretty normal. Dropping into a couple of employment agencies helps you learn what the correct colors to wear are for that particular time period. Smelling of a nice shower is a good strategy as well. Now you have them interested, especially if you have brushed your teeth and can smile and pretend you are normal. I have practiced deep breathing and biting my tongue during interviews.

One time, just after I had my last psychotic break back in 1985, I found myself again looking for a job which was a vital necessity since I was a single mom of a seven-year-old son. I was on my way to a temporary staffing agency that had advertised for a memory writer operator, a particular skill I had acquired, and I began shivering from the cold. I had left the house without a coat, not realizing it was a cold November day. The bright idea of ducking into a store in Manhattan and buying myself a nice warm coat with my trusty credit card occurred to me. When I got to the agency, I looked very normal. Had I walked in on that cold day without a coat, the interview would have been a failure. People tend to notice things like that and since their livelihood depends on their decisions, it is good to get them to think that you are normal. Who would guess that only a few weeks before voices were talking to me from out of space and from the radio? That was thirty-six years ago and my last psychotic episode. I avoided hospitalization then by going to the pharmacy and filling a renewal on my prescription. I did this after my seven-year-old son cooked a bowl of rice for his mother who was in a psychotic stupor. I learned to take my medicine.

That interview netted me a stint working for a group of psychiatrists for a prominent health care center as a transcriber of dictation tapes. Pretending I was normal indeed was tested to the limit at this place, but I had the advantage of having firsthand knowledge of all the psychiatric psychobabble. Also, by transcribing the tapes day in and day out, I came to realize that there are very many people with psychiatric problems in New York City alone. I am fully aware that I am not the only one struggling to maintain my homeostasis.

Another major strength that I have developed is keeping my mouth shut. I have the right to remain silent. Sometimes it is appropriate to simply nod and smile at just the right moment and not say what you are thinking. I did get fired from more than one job before I developed this strength. Not grinning can be an asset as well (again with the tongue-biting). You need to develop a keen sense of observation and notice what the other people are doing. If they are all busy working, you might as well plow in and be productive. On one job, I did not have the foggiest notion of what to do, so I just spread out all the papers with questions around about the ledge that surrounded my desk. I then waited for the lawyer I had just been hired to work for to answer those questions. But he didn't know most of the answers either, so the papers just lay neatly surrounding my desk for a long while.

Pretending you are normal is not all that easy. You need to develop self-control and restraint. If you do that long enough, you end up more normal than the rest of the population.

This begs the question: why pretend to be something that you are not? It is OK not to be normal, and in fact we are all unique. But the real question is who will take care of you if you do not take care of yourself? *I am normal for me.* Being gainfully employed paid my rent, gave me freedom from psych wards, and allowed me to live in society. I do believe that work for me was occupational therapy. It forced me to act normal daily. But, if I were hired as a handicapped employee, my take-home pay would more than likely be far less.

An important strength I have learned is to take my medicine. I might have avoided many breakdowns had I learned this earlier. However, in my defense I must add that I take the smallest dose possible of perphenazine. Had I allowed myself to be treated with the elephantine dosages of medicine first introduced that turned me into a zombie and then a human pretzel, I would be a shadow of myself. So, although I went through a lot of suffering before I realized I had to take my medicine, I am happy that I decided finally to do it on my own terms. If you can pretend you are normal without medicine — and that includes the self-prescribed illegal ones, or alcohol — then bravo to you.

The major source of my ability to be sane again of course is the decision to believe in Jesus Christ as my Lord and Savior. The Holy Bible is my roadmap to living. This way I can be in a crazy world but not be of the craziness.

By applying Bible principles, I have a plan I can follow. In the morning I get up and have learned to begin my daily battle by sending up my praises and thanksgiving to Almighty God. I wondered what some battle thousands of years ago as recorded in the Old Testament of the Bible has to do with my present-day life and realized that it makes sense to put the Lord first in my day. After a great deal of pondering and plaintive, fervent praying, it became clear that all the battles won by the Israelites had begun by praising the Lord and putting Him first. I learned to put on my Ephesians' Armor every day (Ephesians 6:10-18), and I do not go out without my spiritual protection. My motto is to do the best that I can and then the next day, I do the same thing all over again. By spending time in prayer and meditation when on a bus or other transportation, I am relaxed and composed. I ask God to send His angels ahead of me to order my day. My supervisor on the job I held for more than ten years wrote on my performance review that I am indispensable! I know this is flattery, but I like it anyway. It made me feel secure and feeling secure is a good thing.

I put God in charge of my finances. I had a good job, so I could afford to tithe and give offerings. I am debt-free, I always have money in my pocket, and I have everything I need. My cup is not half-empty; my cup is not half-full; my cup is full and running over (See: Psalm 23). As the saying goes, "God has turned my stumbling blocks into steppingstones!"

One of the things I learned in life by coping with my mental chemical imbalance challenge is that it is OK not to be perfect. After all, when I read in Revelations that all of heaven was quiet for a very long time waiting for the one who is perfect and the only one who was ever perfect (See: Rev. 5:1-14), I am relieved to realize it didn't have to be me. Jesus Christ has already filled this position. Being perfect is just too hard, but being the best I can be is possible for me. What a relief that the price for all my imperfections has been paid and I have the right to boldly access the Throne of Grace [See: Hebrews 4:16].

Sometimes I have mood swings and feel fearful, doubtful, or suspicious. Sometimes I stuff my feelings with food. I can bring all these sometimes moments to the Lord and ask Him to help me deal with them. If I remember to do that, I can continue in my role as a normal person who bears the responsibility of being a representative of my Divine Savior. That means I must watch my conduct.

I must watch my mouth. Am I lying or gossiping? Am I feeling jealous or eating compulsively? If so, then it is time to repent. And then I remember it is not about my perfection but about the perfection of Jesus Christ.

I like to keep an attitude of gratitude. When I think of all I have, then it is easy. I can walk. I have sight, hearing, good sense (and even a little nonsense). My son is a fine young man and I am enormously proud of him. I have good friends from church and close personal friends. I do not drive. I am convinced that handling heavy equipment is out of the question for me, so I have never driven a car. I can walk! Other people drive me places and I reciprocate by buying them gas or taking my drivers out to eat. This is my contribution to making the planet greener and safer.

I can be grateful for my chemical imbalance because it has made me more compassionate of others. Whatever my path has been, it has led me to the path of following the Lord and experiencing His mercy and compassion. I am not quick to judge because I do not want others to judge me, and anyway, the Good Book tells me not to do that [See: Matthew 7:1-2].

Now that I have asked Jesus Christ into my heart and invited Him to be my Lord and Savior, I carry His Holy Spirit with me. What could be more exciting than a relationship with the Creator of the Universe?

When arguments arise over the Bible, I find my bearings by remembering the Greatest Commandment [See: Matthew 22: 36-40]. It really is very brilliant. I must

Love God with my whole heart, my whole mind, my whole soul, and all my strength and love others as myself. Loving myself makes me capable of loving others. And loving others as I love myself is the best way to obey God and show our love to Him.

The challenge arises because sometimes there are days when I do not like myself and other days when people violate my boundaries, which provokes me. But aha, as I read further in the Bible, I am instructed to pray for my enemies. For some reason, when I do this, it diffuses the tension of conflict that throws me into frenzy. And when the enemy of God attacks me with negativity, I draw close to Jesus and let Him fight my battles for me. Jesus is my shield.

I have learned that the word of God of the Holy Bible strengthens me. I have learned that *"the joy of the Lord is my strength"* [Nehemiah 8:10]. If my joy dissipates, I can focus on the words of David in Psalms where he writes, *"Restore the joy of your salvation"* [Psalm 51:12]. When I dwell on the awesomeness of the gift of salvation, my joy always returns.

Finally, I have learned that although I cannot fix me, the indwelling Holy Spirit of God is ever bringing healing to me.

Who needs a word of encouragement today? Is it the little baby just learning to walk? Is it the toddler struggling to learn both English and Spanish? How brave of that toddler to tackle so much work! Is it the student on the bus who worries about the future? Is it the elderly man hobbling down the street who needs just a smile? Let us encourage one another and never have the time or inclination to kick someone when they are down. If we all go around encouraging each other, there will be no wars.

I am a witness to the love and mercy of Our Lord. Yes, I still have hang-ups. I am not sinless, but I do sin less. I now understand that sitting with pain is crucial to my recovery. I am learning to bear up with my feelings and refuse to run away from them. I learned that feelings are not always facts. Yes, at times I still stuff my feelings down with food and try to sweeten life up with sugary concoctions, but I have been marijuana- and nicotine-free for over almost eighteen years since I rededicated my life to Christ. I look forward still to further healing. I am confident that the Holy Spirit leads and guides me and that the process of healing is continuing as I am being sanctified.

I experience the joy of the Lord daily. I look forward to further recovery and being propelled into the purposes of helping establish God's kingdom here on Earth. It is exciting trusting in the Lord, and I believe. I understand that the purpose of my pain is for me to help in the healing of others who are suffering and to point them to the love and mercy of Jesus.

This verse comes up in my spirit:

> *But, as it is written: Eye hath not seen, nor ear heard, neither have entered into the heart of man, the things which God hath prepared for them that love Him. But God hath revealed them unto us by His Spirit: for the Spirit searches all things, yea, the deep things of God.* [I Corinthians 2:9-10]

So now you see I really am normal for me. I exist; therefore, God exists. Look at your own life and see if you come to the same conclusion.

THE PRESENT

I like the radio jingle that I heard announcing, "Every day is a present that we open, and that's why we call it the present."

Now I have retired and reached my seventy-second birthday. I help with my darling granddaughter and enjoy living in the suburbs. Yes, there are still things that hurt, such as the death of a friend or a friend having difficulties. But I realize that God never promised that we would not have troubles. He did, however, promise that He would always be there to help us through the troubles of life. And He is faithful to that promise to those who believe and trust in Him.

When I was fifty-seven, I realized I had no savings for my retirement. I prayed about that and shortly after found a very rewarding position in a corporation that valued its employees. I retired comfortably just in time to help take care of my granddaughter who was then six months old. Now she is four!

I never imagined how wonderful it would be to take care of that little one and how much I could love her. I thoroughly enjoy all her milestones and being a positive influence in her life. Now we read, sing, do jigsaw puzzles, play with Play-Doh and glitter, finger paint and watercolor, run, and play hide and seek. I am having the time of my life! I have so much to look forward to and so much to enjoy right now. Tall trees envelop our large back yard where I play with my son's dog and reminisce about how I enjoyed a similar little area enveloped by trees as a very young child.

For most of my life I lived in an urban community. So, when my son told me his plan to buy a home in the suburbs with an apartment for me, I hesitated for a moment. I always considered myself a city person. I did not know if I could adjust to the slower pace of the suburbs. However, it occurred to me that if I didn't take up my son's offer, distance would separate us and I would not have the opportunity to see him and my little granddaughter as much as if I lived in his house. So, a little over two years ago, I made a major change in my life.

It was a big ordeal deciding what to take and what to give up. I prayed for guidance as to what to give away and what to take with me. In the end, I filled an entire Salvation Army truck with all the things I was not taking with me. And there was not even room in the truck for another chair.

Interestingly, I find living out in the suburbs very agreeable to me. The trees and the fresh air invigorate me. I love the bird population and their songs. I am enthralled when I see the deer! The area is very picturesque, and I frequently feel as if I have stepped into a Thomas Kinkade picture. Beauty surrounds me and I love my environment. And, of course I love being around my little granddaughter and family.

The house my son bought is close to a nice Bible-believing church and I have been welcomed there. It is just a ten-minute walk from my home. Since I do not drive, on days when there is ice and snow or in the evening when it is dark, there is always someone there kind enough to drive me back and forth to church. I attend church, Bible classes, prayer meetings, and other events. My walk with the Lord is getting closer every day. I am happy that He has provided a church so close to my new home. I do not miss any of the stuff I gave up and am quite comfortable. I have everything I need!

At another church a town away, I found a group called Celebrate Recovery. I attend meetings there every week to help me learn to turn my hurts, hang-ups, and habits over to the Lord instead of stuffing my feelings with food. My recovery is slow and arduous. But, for all the chaos I went through in my early life, I think I am doing very well, and I have hope that I can break bad food habits that no longer serve me.

I have time to reflect every day on the wonders of the Lord who delivered me from so much self-sabotage in the past. I pray every day for guidance and direction, wisdom, and the empowerment of the Holy Spirit to lead and guide me. I pray for other people and for the establishment of God's kingdom here on Earth. As the song goes, "Every day with the Lord is Sweeter than the Day Before."

I have learned a winning strategy to help me out of down-day funks. I focus on the Bible verse that states, *"The Joy of the Lord is my strength"* (Nehemiah 8:10). I realize that the enemy of God is out to steal the strength of those who follow Christ, so of course he would set traps to rob us of our joy. When I reflect on the marvelous gift of salvation, I find my joy returns. What a joy it is to know that my name is written in the Book of Life! If I feel unloved, I focus on the love of Jesus Christ.

By having the Holy Bible as my compass, I find it helps me bear with the problems that go on in the world. It is true that much is written in the Bible to warn us of the tribulations of life. But I cling to the cross of Christ, to Him, and to the power of His Resurrection and our atonement through His precious blood. I depend on the guidance of the Holy Spirit. I find the power to keep my heart and mind on the Lord and not worry about those things that must occur before Jesus returns to the Earth again, as it is prophesized.

It is difficult writing about the past, but I am propelled to do so with the hope that my writing will illuminate the way for someone else to be able to come to the light of Jesus. I hope to encourage those who are already in the light to continue growing in the knowledge, mercy, and grace of the Lord.

It occurs to me that had I been successful in my earlier attempts to end my life, I would have missed it all. I would have missed motherhood, the wonderful friendships I enjoy both in the past and the present, and the thrill of being a grandmother. I have a deep gratitude that my Heavenly Father rescued me from my own self-destruction and despair, picked me up, cleaned me up, and turned me around. Yes, every day is a present!

As the world reels from COVID-19, I find myself somewhat prepared by the life I have lived to cope with what is happening. Yet who could be prepared to deal with this pandemic? Underneath it all, I have had this deep-rooted feeling that the other shoe would always drop but I never expected it to drop on the whole world. So far, I have not been anywhere for more than three months. My days are passing quickly. My little granddaughter keeps me busy and literally hopping! It is wonderful that I am here to watch her while her parents attend to their jobs which they can easily perform from home. I am aware that while we are all in the same storm, we are not all in the same boat. Thinking about it, I am on the Good Ship Lollipop. My granddaughter and I play the different roles from the video of *The Hobbit*. I get to be the Goblin King, or Frodo. She plays the role of Bilbo Baggins. To make it more fun, her parents ordered the Bilbo cape along with the light-up sword named Sting. My granddaughter gets limits of a half hour television each in the morning and after nap. We have watched *The Hobbit* as well as *The Lord of the Rings*, *The Wizard of Oz*, *Ben and Holly*, and *Peppa Pig*. I constantly lose at Zingo and Kids on Stage. We get to practice some chess and chess puzzles. Of course, there is racing in the yard, bubble stuff, and balloons, and we make batter and bake cornbread up in my apartment.

The last time I was out, other than taking a walk around the area where I live, was when I went to my pastor's mother's wake on March 12. By then the noise of the pandemic was in the air. I hesitated about going to the wake but the friend who drove me is a retired nurse who seemed confident that it was all right for us to go. At that time, I had not quite grasped the phrase "social distancing." We paid our respects and hugged and kissed a few people. I talked with my pastor's fourteen-year-old son who has Down's syndrome. He was handling the passing of his grandmother as well as he could. As always, being around him uplifted me. He told me, "Sometimes I am up and sometimes I am down." I complimented him on his honesty and told him that the angels were watching over him. As we got ready to leave, I offered to take my friend out for a bite to eat. We went to a nearby crowded diner. We had a good time and she drove me home.

The next day, my son called me on his speaker phone from his car as he traveled to his job in New York City. He told me he was taking my granddaughter out of pre-K so that she would not bring home the virus to me. I told him I was afraid to be the one who would give it to her. He insisted that I was the one who was at risk because of my age and the fact that I have asthma. Of course, I am happy to be taking care of my granddaughter, so it is no real sacrifice to give up my time at the Y and the senior center. Little did I know that I would also end up giving up church, Bible study, and in-person prayer meetings. I am doing my best to adjust to the same thing that everyone in the world is confronted with. I wonder when will this be over and how best to use the time of isolation. So far, I have been spending the time that I am not taking care of my granddaughter in prayer and amassing information. For diversion, I have my online chess games, Zoom meetings, reading, social media, and my writing.

Yes, we are in a battle with an unseen enemy. But in my world view, that has always been the case. An evil has manifested itself throughout the entire world.

My situation in this pandemic is somewhat ideal. I live in my son's house in a separate apartment. I am not completely alone because I am attending to my little granddaughter. I am retired and have no job security to fret about. I have food on order with an internet delivery service. I have everything I need but my heart breaks for those who don't.

It is difficult to feel the joy of the Lord while your heart is breaking. But deep down, I have the faith that tells me, *"And we know that all things work together for good to them that love God, to them who are the called according to his purpose"* [Romans 8:28]. I am praying fervently for a miracle. I pray that hearts will turn to the Lord. Where else is there to turn to?

I walk around the neighborhood for as long as a half hour without seeing a moving car. It is spring, the birds are singing, the trees are splendidly dressed, and the weather is lovely. I suppose under these circumstances it is ordinary that the whole pandemic seems unreal. I spent the first two weeks at home thinking that the plague would soon go away, that it was all just a hoax. Now I am prepared to stay home for as long as it takes. I am calm but mourn over the devastation that the pandemic has caused. I must limit my time listening to the news to avoid feeling too sad, but my curiosity keeps me up to date.

A few weeks before we started social distancing, my primary care physician told me he wanted me to see a psychiatrist. He wanted to be sure he had prescribed the right psychotropic. So, I met with my new psychiatrist via video conference on my tablet. The visit was all of fifteen minutes and in the end, it seemed I was in better shape than him. In addition to his video consultations, he is on the front lines treating patients in the emergency room. He told me I looked and sounded normal and should stick with the medication I am taking.

I do not expect very much from psychiatrists. They are all too busy to spend time with a well patient. I saw one a couple of years ago who would spend twenty minutes with me, but I had to wait five hours in his waiting room. It is a good thing I only need to check in with them to maintain the medication that I have been taking for over thirty-five years.

I find friendship much more rewarding than going to a psychiatrist. It is extremely difficult to find a psychiatrist who is not in it apparently just for the money. In my experience, patients are routinely overdosed with psychotropics to keep them manageable and to cause the least bit of work. Realizing that the pandemic will lead to people dealing with extreme anxieties and that they will encounter a general unconcern from the psychiatric community really peeves me. So even though I know it is not fair to paint all psychiatrists with the same brush, not only do I deal with fears, I deal with anger and of course sadness over all the suffering going on in the world.

I have Zoom meetings during the lockdown with my Celebrate Recovery group, but my emotional overeating persists despite all the attention I have been giving it. Admittedly, the food obsession has been with me for a long time.

I have a Bible study Zoom meeting on Monday nights and a Zoom meeting with the prayer team from my church on Wednesday nights. Saturday mornings is a telephone prayer meeting with my accountability partner from Celebrate Recovery. Sunday, I go to YouTube and access my Sunday service that way. A friend at church delivers the communion elements to my rural mailbox. I am not confident to return to face-to-face meetings.

The possibility of me bringing COVID-19 home to my family frightens me. My plan is as things open up, I will stay right here on my Good Ship Lollipop until I feel confident enough to return to the swim of life.

Fortunately, I have my relationship with Jesus Christ to help me through my hurdles. I know that I am a work in progress and I claim the Bible verse that states, *"And I am certain that God, who began the good work within you, will continue his work until it is finally finished on the day when Christ Jesus returns* [Philippians 1:6 (NLT)]. An incident that occurred when I was just ten years old pops up in my mind. I was having a great two-week time at Camp Trinity. I had been cast in a part for a play about the seasons of the year. My part represented winter. I was to come on stage at the cue of "the snow is falling," get to the center of the stage, and plop down as if I were the snow. The part thrilled me. However, on the night of the play, my cue was not read, and I was left out. I cried my heart out. Somehow that incident seemed to sum up my life as I knew it up to that point in time. The grief of being left out of my family and shunted around like I did not matter poured out of me as I sobbed uncontrollably. I finally got my composure back, but I bring the incident up to reflect on how much healing I have had in life. I do have a purpose. I am part of the Divine Plan. I realize this now as it is written: *And he said unto me, "It is done. I am Alpha and Omega, the beginning and the end. I will give unto him that is athirst of the fountain of the water of life freely"* [Revelation 21.6].

The murder of George Floyd provoking demonstrations where some turned to riots brought back many memories for me. One memory is that before I retired, I contemplated moving to South Carolina to be near my niece. I relayed my idea to her. She told me, "Well you know, Auntie Renie, if you move here you must go to the white church." What is wrong with that picture? Apartheid in the Christian church must be anathema to the Lord, for it is written in John 17:20-21:

> [20] *Neither pray I for these alone, but for them also which shall believe on me through their word:* [21]*that they all may; as thou Father, art in me, and I in thee, that they also may be one in us; that the world may believe that thou hast sent me.*

It occurs to me that it must displease the Lord greatly for the body of Christ to have such disunity. How can we profess to love God who we cannot see if we cannot love those we can see? [Based on 1 John 4:20].

If anyone doubts that we are all given the opportunity for salvation, please turn to the following vision of heaven in the Bible verse located at Revelation 7:9-10:

> *9 After this I beheld, and, lo, a great multitude which no man could number, of all nations, and kindreds and people and tongues, stood before the throne and before the Lamb, clothed with white robes, and palms in their hands. 10 And cried with a loud voice, saying, Salvation to our God which sitteth upon the throne, and unto the Lamb.*

I doubt that anyone who harbors racism in their heart would be comfortable in heaven; I doubt if they could get there without repentance.

Now, it is early June and things are beginning to open up. I pray that the Spirit of God unites our hearts so we can leave a better world to our progeny. We will see what the rest of 2020 looks like. May the grace, mercy, and love of our Lord Jesus be with you.

GRATITUDE

I am thankful for my salvation, that God loved me so much that He sent His only son to redeem me. I am thankful for Jesus Christ my Lord and Savior. I am thankful for God's forgiveness, His mercy, and His grace. I am thankful for the precious blood of Christ that cleanses me from my sins, and I am thankful for the friends who God has sent on my path during my life. I am thankful that God has kept me alive through many of my own self-destructive acts. I am thankful for the Holy Spirit who leads and guides me through the minefields of life. I am thankful for my sisters and brothers in Christ who have encouraged me and help me grow in the knowledge of the Lord.

I am thankful for the Bible which is my compass and GPS. I am thankful that I have time for reflection and devotion. I am thankful for the hope of everlasting life.

I thank God I live in a country that allows me to find Bible-believing churches. I thank the Good Lord for including me as part of the family of God and welcoming me into the Body of Christ. I thank Jesus for the blood He shed for me on the cross.

I am thankful for the twelve step programs of Overeaters Anonymous and Adult Children of Alcoholics. I am thankful for finding the group Celebrate Recovery which adapts the twelve steps to the Christian Beatitudes. I am thankful that God has provided programs to help me heal and I am particularly thankful for the recovery I received while attending Solid Foundation Ministry; there I learned to forgive not only others but also to forgive myself and to turn to the Bible for help, stability, and healing.

I am very thankful for the wonderful son that God has blessed me with and my son's wonderful wife who birthed my beautiful, intelligent grandchild.

I am thankful for all the good people who encouraged me along the way, and I am thankful that I decided to be like them rather than like people who are hurtful. I am thankful that I know enough to pray for hurtful people who have not yet decided to be kind.

I am thankful for my sanity. When I stand at a bus stop, I thank God that I can figure out which bus to take. I am thankful that I live in a time in history where there are medications that help with chemical imbalance issues. I am thankful for having the humility to accept I must take medication. I am thankful that I am alive and well and God's Holy Spirit lives within me

I am thankful for a normal day.

I am thankful for the gifts of health, sight, hearing, and compassion.

And yes, I am thankful for my toes and fingers!

Every day is Thanksgiving!

Abba Father, Alleluia!

ABBA FATHER

Father God, You are so good to me. Your compassion is beyond compare. Your mercy has provided for my redemption through the precious blood of Jesus' sacrifice on the cross. Your benevolent love has washed my sins and trespasses against You from my soul. You are so loving and gracious. I know it is true that God is love. You are truly a gracious, loving Father.

Father, I was so lost in my sin and rebellion but instead of punishing me, You showed me mercy and grace. You delivered me from my wickedness and forgave me of my sins. You washed me in the precious blood of Jesus. Daily I turn to You in gratitude all the days of my life. I love You and adore You. You are a good Father and have shown me Your love. Help me through the guidance of Your Holy Spirit to be the person you created me to be.

Father God, You know the desires of my heart and I trust You to know what is good for me even when I do not know what is good for me. I love You and adore You and ask that You keep me on the path of righteousness all the days of my life through Jesus Christ my Lord and Savior.

There were times when I rebelled because I erroneously believed You had abandoned me. As I reflect over the period in my life when my faith and trust were so weak that I turned toward things that I knew were in opposition to Your will, I see Your divine mercy in knowing my sin-sick soul was stumbling. You were there at all times to prevent me from dying in my sin. Father, You know me and my weaknesses, and I trust You. I have decided to follow Jesus all the days of my life. I trust You to keep me on the path of righteousness and to hold me.

I am so blessed to have known Your precious presence in my life. You have encouraged me and shown me Your love. You have made known to me the reality of your existence. I see You have always been there for me. You have shown me mercy in forgiving my sins committed through ignorance and outright rebellion. Father God, I am forever indebted to You for putting up with my ignorance. I trust You to fill me with a spirit of wisdom and to lead and guide me continually through Jesus, my Lord, and Savior and to continue to fill me with Your Holy Spirit.

Abba Father, You are the Most High God. There is none like You. You are the Creator of the universe and everything in it. There is nothing too difficult for You. Father God, I commit myself to serving You. I thank you for Your provision of Your precious son, Jesus, to give me a hope to approach Your throne of grace knowing that by His precious blood I am washed clean of all my sins. I thank You for providing me with the wisdom of Your Holy Spirit indwelling me, leading and guiding me in the process of becoming who You created me to be.

As I look around my life daily, I am amazed at Your loving kindness and mercy to me. I am forever grateful that You have touched my hand and led me back home to You. I am still sorry for all the rebellious acts I made toward You and would rather have trusted and obeyed You from the beginning of my life. Yet I am thankful that my suffering led me to You. You have given me the desires of my heart and I trust You to continue to do that. And my desire is to improve on my ability to love You in greater capacity evermore. I thank You for Your divine revelation and I pray for a steadfast spirit.

You are a God of truth. There is no falsehood in You, and You cannot tolerate falsehood. I am sorry for all the times I pretended I was OK when I was not because that was a lie. Your enemy is a liar, and I was like him before I received Your mercy and grace. As I come closer to You, I am even more aware of all that is false in me and I renounce that falsehood and ask You to lead me to a life of integrity.

Father God, You alone are faithful to Your word. Your word is always truth. I may not always be happy with the truth, but nonetheless I recognize the truth is the only right way. You have left me to my own devices and let me suffer the consequences of falsehood, so I learned that Your way alone is the right way. Thank you, Father; You have washed me in the blood of Jesus. Your way is truth, love, and peace.

Lord God, You are mighty and reign in heaven above all the Earth. The angels and all those who perceive You adore You. You are responsible for all the galaxies and the motions of the planets and the fabric they sit in. Yet You are in the details of each and every one of our lives. You are the Mighty God, and it is my pleasure to serve You. I ask only that You make the direction in my life clear to me so that I may be a worthwhile daughter.

So many times, You have shown me Your grace and mercy. When my soul was dulled by poor decisions and sins of disobedience, You revealed your mighty love to me and I am honored to be so blessed. I cannot count the answered prayers that You have blessed me with. Lord, You have blessed me with all I need to live a life of peace and love and to follow You. I ask only that my light reflects Your glory to draw others to You. What a mighty God you are.

There is no prayer that is worthy of Your awesomeness. Who could comprehend Your great love? Who could comprehend Your divine intelligence, mercy, faithfulness, beauty, and most of all holiness? I look forward to spending all eternity surrounded by Your unimaginable love. You are worthy, Lord, of all praises, honor, and glory. It is with humble gratitude that I appreciate the honor of learning to serve You.

Holy, Holy, Holy is the Lord God Almighty. You are worthy of worship and praise. By Your might You have created all things. Father God, I am forever thankful for Your grace, love and mercy. I thank You for the Holy Spirit teaching, leading, and guiding me. I thank You for sending Your only son to die on the cross whom You raised from the dead so that anyone who believes would find forgiveness of sins and the everlasting hope of spending eternity in heaven with You. Thank You, Father.

Father God, I thank You for your sacred Word, Jesus Christ, my Lord and Savior. What love and mercy You displayed by offering Your son Jesus to be a finished work of Your divine love and sending us Your Holy Spirit to dwell in us, leading and guiding us all the days of our life. Your mercy is unfathomable. When I look back over my life, I realize You were always there. Though my heart was seared with resentments and anger, You delivered me and kept me throughout my life. I love You Lord, and ask only that You help me love You more.

Father, You are the Everlasting God. You always were and always will be. You wrap your creation in Your eternal love, and I am part of Your creation. I now understand that You have always been in my life even when I was unaware. Father, forgive my oversight and ignorance of Your eternal love. I pray and ask You to help me assist others in becoming aware of the one true Everlasting God, the Father, the Son, and the Holy Spirit.

Thank You for sending your Holy Spirit to assist and comfort me in my daily walk with You. I have received so much healing of all the hurts and confusions I encountered in life. Your grace and mercy saved me with the precious blood of Jesus. Your love is beyond expression but is shown by your love, grace, and mercy. All honor and glory is due to you, Abba Father.

In my own lack of vision, I did not understand how much love You had for me. Much of my mental anguish was brought on by neglect of those who were assigned to nurture me. I see now that You were always there and saw when I needed help. Only because You revealed your enormous love am I able to begin to grasp Your infinite wisdom. I pray that through the message revealed in the mess You brought me out of that others will recognize that You truly are the God who sees all.

Father, I heard your Holy Spirit encouraging me and promising to strengthen me. I wondered why I needed to be so strong. Then, life unfolded and I needed the strength You promised. True to Your word, You provided that strength. Indeed, my strength is only through You. You are the rock of my salvation and I am forever thankful for Your provision of strength. Day by day, every minute, every hour, You are near me. You are a friend closer than a brother. Your Holy Spirit leads and guides me. Your word is truth.

Let us praise, honor, and give glory to the God who is with us. Father, You know my deepest and most secret thoughts. You show me the answers to questions I have not even asked out loud or in the silence of my soul. I know that You are with me.

God Almighty, You have provided me with all that I need. In all my anxieties and worries, You have always been God Almighty, the lover and caretaker of my soul. The very fact that I am alive and well and that Your Holy Spirit leads and guides me is evidence that You are God Almighty. It is true that You are love and You are wonderful in providing Your beloved son, Jesus, to me and others. Father God, you are outstanding!

www.ingramcontent.com/pod-product-compliance
Lightning Source LLC
LaVergne TN
LVHW091548060526
838200LV00036B/750